BORN TO DIE?

MARY BUTLER

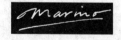

FOR DENISE

With thanks to:

Mrs Boyle

Barbara and Joe

Marie Therese

Evelyn

Nollaig

Paula

Chris and Sue

Marion

For their kind permission to reprint their letters

First published in 1995 by
Marino Books
An imprint of Mercier Press
16 Hume Street Dublin 2

Trade enquiries to Mercier Press
PO Box 5, 5 French Church Street,
Cork

A Marino Original

© Mary Butler 1995

ISBN 1 86023 009 1

10 9 8 7 6 5 4 3 2 1

A CIP record for this title is available
from the British Library

Cover design by Niamh Sharkey from
family photographs
Set by Richard Parfrey in Caslon
Regular 9.5/15 and Avant Garde
Printed in Ireland by ColourBooks,
Baldoyle Industrial Estate, Dublin 13

CONTENTS

Medical description of James's condition by Professor E. J. Guiney of Our Lady's Hospital for Sick Children, Crumlin

Baby James Boyle was born on 21 January 1988 with a major complex congenital abnormality of great rarity. The incidence of the abnormality which James had at birth would be of the order of one in fifty thousand births. The medical terminology for the condition is a Cloacal Exstrophy. In this abnormality the lower half of the baby's anterior abdominal wall is defective and the baby is born with its urinary bladder and the lower portion of its bowel protruding through the defect in the abdominal wall. It is exceptional for infants with this condition to survive, though some have done so. Following major reconstructive surgery, undertaken over a number of years, those individuals who have survived have done so with very significant physical disability, particularly affecting the control of their bladder and back passage, as a consequence of which they are incontinent of both urine and faeces.

Shortly after his birth Baby James had an initial surgery to reconstruct the lower portion of his bowel and to establish a colostomy. This stabilised the situation and although he never thrived physically a further major operation was undertaken in August 1988, aimed at reconstructing his bladder. This procedure posed too great a challenge for Baby James's physical reserves and he died shortly after the operation.

FOREWORD

After James's death, and even before it, I had to ask myself the question 'Why did it happen?' Could something have been done differently? I have no doubt these questions went through Mary and Rick's minds as well.

James's death left me afraid and angry, shocked and frustrated. Being a priest and living in Rome, I had no one to talk to. This heightened my sense of isolation and, because Mary and Rick were the first couple I married just after my ordination, the death of their child raised sizeable personal questions for me.

I still remember the day Mary and I went to the hospital and as I write this I can still hear James's cries. He seemed to know that the arrival of the nurse meant more pain and distress for him and there was nothing, but nothing I could do to alleviate his pain.

Afterwards we went for a drink and Mary told me the whole story of James's birth, and the question of the sex of the child. She also expressed her hopes for James if he were to come through his illness. I remember the fears she had for him that he might be isolated and bullied at school or that he would find it personally and psychologically very difficult to carry with him through life the obvious disabilities he would always have. I remember the way the conversation oscillated between hopes and dreams of how things might be, and then the quiet prayer that maybe it would be best if God took him now; and then the anger towards a God who would allow such a small innocent child to suffer for something that he never did.

Early on the morning of James's funeral I went out to the hospital morgue to pray beside his coffin. My attempts to enter the morgue were frustrated because it was locked and I had to go and get an attendant with a key. While that was going on some members of the family, including Mary and Rick, arrived. I remember the funeral liturgy with the chaplain and the burial in the graveyard – a grave which now embraces not only James but both his maternal grandparents as well. I also recall the bravery of Mary and Rick in the face of James's death. One of the things I found difficult was that the anger I felt inside at God was something that, if they did share it, they did not express outwardly. I also felt very sad – sad in particular for both of them, because the hopes and dreams that they had had would never now be realised. Added to this was a sense of frustration because, as a priest, I was supposed to be supportive and strong and not to be grieving. Yet, inwardly, I was shattered. The God I believe in is an all-kind, all-loving, all-merciful God and I could not square that concept of God with the death of James.

I found it very hard to have hope at that time. Every morning since I was small I was taught to say an Act of Hope, Faith and Charity. On the day of James's death and the day of his funeral I did not say an Act of Hope. And yet I realise that without hope, without faith and without a belief in the resurrection, life would, in many ways, be meaningless.

Even while I was in the seminary I was interested in the topic of death. I wrote about it for my BD thesis and I studied the theology of the last things: death, judgement, heaven and hell. But while able, in an academic manner, to treat of these topics, the concrete reality of this death brought home to me the true meaning of what I had studied intellectually for some years. I don't have the answers; I don't know. While most people do not seem to think much about death I guess I live in the constant presence of the inevitability of it. The fact is that I am sometimes haunted by the terrifying possibility of total extinction.

I had learnt that death is life's greatest possibility. But with James I came face-to-face with the fact that while all other responsibilities can be transferred or avoided or at least shared, we all face death alone. James faced death alone.

I honestly do not think you get over death. Time heals, they say. I am not sure I agree. What time grants you is the ability to go on, to carry on with life despite the traumatic death which occurred in the past. Time and time again I have met people who have recounted the last hours, the last minutes, the last seconds of somebody's mortal life. Why they go into so much detail and how they remember the experience so vividly I do not know. What I do know is that slowly, very slowly, people get used to the reality that someone they love is no longer there. I think the pain stays with them. It is not lifted but you learn to go on in life carrying that pain. In fact it becomes such a part of you that it is hard to imagine life without it.

As a Christian and a priest I believe that death is not the end, rather that it is only the beginning of a new and eternal existence. For a long time after James's death I sought some reason, some rationale behind his life, his suffering and his death. I never found it. The best analogy that I found is that of life as a tapestry. If you look at the front of a tapestry you see how each thread plays its part in the building up of a masterpiece, a work of art. Although many thousands of threads are used of many different colours, each one augments the work. Each one has its place no matter how long or how short. The tapestry is beautiful viewed from the front but if you go round the back you find, instead of the clear, beautiful picture, a rough impression of the true image. Jagged threads of different lengths stick out, apparently at random. Maybe, just maybe, we look at the tapestry of life from the wrong side.

I think with James's death I came to realise that the more you love, the more you are confronted with death, but his death left me with a sensation of bewilderment and denial. There is life and then it is over. Human beings are mortal and we all die. It is, after all, the only thing we know for certain about our future. Yes, of course, death is a natural event, but it cannot and should not happen to a little child, I said to myself; it's impossible; it's incredible.

Another difficulty was that in our society it is not the thing for a priest to grieve publicly and yet how could I preach a loving God with my lips while cursing him in my heart? While feeling a sense of rage and rebellion within my own self I kept asking the question: why did he die when he was so young, so innocent? Why not somebody much older? With his death the abstract theory about everybody dying became a somewhat cruel absurdity. And yet surely none of us has a right to remain here? Had James really disappeared into nothingness? Is death the definite end of the relationship we have with one another? Or is it possible to go beyond the boundaries of death. Ironically, my questioning led, I think, to a deepening of my belief in God and my trust in a life after death. Somehow I came to an understanding also that the experience of love is itself an experience of eternity.

In the end, James's short life and early death challenged me to assert my belief in eternal life, to assert my belief in a loving God, despite the bitterness I felt within and in some ways still feel. I have often said that if ever I sit down and write my autobiography, the subtitle of the book may well be: 'Living with Ambiguity'.

Although I never did, and maybe never could have, resolved the issues which are raised by James, I learnt to keep on going, to keep on searching, to keep on loving and to keep on believing.

Ciaran

1

LABOUR

Several times over the weekend I had said to Rick that I felt 'really pregnant' all of a sudden. I couldn't explain it. I had felt it since the Friday afternoon when I was going round the supermarket. Maybe it was that the baby was getting heavier, I thought. Maybe it was just more discomfort all of a sudden. The baby wasn't due for nearly seven weeks.

On the Saturday evening my father babysat for us and we went to a session of Irish music about two miles from our house. For only the second time the baby gave an enormous kick in response to the music. The first time had been at a carol concert just before Christmas. It was now the middle of January. It must like both types, I thought – Irish and classical!

On the Sunday my neighbour, Margaret, who lived five doors away from us, reiterated her offer to mind Stephen when I went into hospital. It struck me as vaguely odd or coincidental that she should think of what was so much on my mind also. She subsequently told me that she'd noticed the bump had dropped compared with its position when she'd last seen me.

Later that day, without saying anything to anybody, I got out the little brown suitcase that I had used when going into hospital ten months previously for our first baby, Stephen. It was really

Rick's case – he had sometimes used it when he was coming over for the weekend while we were going out with each other. I packed a couple of nighties, towels, a toilet bag and checked where everything else was that I might need in a hurry. I just had a feeling that I might be kept in when I went to the hospital for my routine check-up the next morning. At the same time I kept telling myself that I was being stupid and irrational.

The Monday morning check-up went smoothly. It was only my second visit to the hospital on that pregnancy. I had opted for what's called 'combined care' which meant I went to my own GP for several visits and he checked my weight, blood pressure and so on, and marked up my card for when I went back to the Coombe. Well, correction, it was my third visit if you counted the check-up on my heart that the first doctor I'd seen had insisted upon. I have a slight heart murmur and she said she hadn't liked the sound of it too much. The heart specialist, however, had dismissed it as nothing to worry about.

So there I was in line. The finger-prick blood test showed my iron levels were fine. A nurse then gave me a kicking chart but I was really taken aback when I looked at it – it said to mark down your baby's movements and if you did not feel ten movements over a twelve-hour period to contact the hospital. I knew there had been days when I had barely scraped together ten infinitesimal movements from the time I woke up until the time I went to sleep at night – a stretch of fifteen or sixteen hours. However, I decided that, while I would mention my worry in general to the doctor, I would go home and count again for a few days before panicking.

There was one other factor niggling me. When I'd been expecting Stephen everyone who examined me exclaimed how big he was for my dates. Now I reckoned that he was due two weeks before the date they had given me. In the case of my second pregnancy I deliberately lied about the date – putting it forward by one week, with the idea of working a week longer than I was meant to. Yet no one had said the baby was big for these dates.

I had never before met the doctor, a man, who examined me that morning and I have never met him since. He told me everything seemed fine. I said I was worried because the baby seemed very quiet. He dismissed this: 'Everything seems in order to me,' he said, adding that the second baby always seemed quieter because you were used to the movement. I could see there was little point in arguing so I said nothing more. I am glad now that he didn't listen to me, although it annoyed me at the time, because I am glad that I was not sent for a scan, although ultimately it would not have had any bearing on the end result.

I went on into work that day. I was working 11am–7pm and I worked the next day also. I was relieved when it came time to go home on the Tuesday. I can remember standing up from my desk and feeling the discomfort again and wishing that the next four weeks were over and I was on maternity leave and could rest. I was due a day off the following day anyway.

That Tuesday evening my only sister, Denise, (we have no brothers) phoned me. We're really very close. She knew I was concerned about the lack of kicking. She wanted to know how the check-up had gone. I told her they'd said everything was fine. But even as I spoke to Denise another little voice in my mind was saying – but you may be going into labour later tonight. It's often struck me since how my mind seemed to operate on two levels – the rational (or semi-rational!) surface and the deeper, instinctive, intuitive one.

I said nothing that night to Rick. I knew I had things almost ready to go to hospital. I thought that if it was anything like Stephen I would have hours and hours of niggles ahead of me before anything would happen, if it was going to happen at all.

But as I lay in bed that night, I did have to admit to myself that it was more than just discomfort now, that I could not go on like this for another six weeks. I didn't sleep well but I dozed on and off.

When I got up the next morning I had a 'show' and the niggles were continuing. With Stephen I had had a show in the morning and he had been born that evening. I told Rick and he said he would stay at home with me if I wanted but he had an important meeting to go to which could possibly go on all day. So I said he should go because I could always get in touch with him if I really needed to.

I suppose as things were so ahead of time I should really have contacted the hospital for advice but that did not occur to me, or to Rick. I was far more preoccupied with the memory of going in with Stephen and, after pains on and off for about nine hours, being categorically told that I was not in labour. This time I was determined not to go near the hospital too soon.

It was my sister's birthday, that day – Wednesday, 20 January.

I went down to Margaret's house to tell her I might need to take her up on her offer of minding Stephen sooner than expected. She wasn't there but her husband, Don, was.

Stephen was starting a cold and was not in good form. He was at the runny nose stage. It suited us both for me to walk up and down with him in my arms for most of the morning. The niggles were no worse but they were still there. While I was walking from sitting-room to kitchen and back again Don called back down to me to see how I was feeling. I was quite cheerful and assured him I'd come down if I needed anything.

Eventually Stephen went up to his cot and had a nap. While he was asleep both Margaret and Don called down to me. We agreed we'd keep in touch and when they'd gone I finished getting my case ready.

The early afternoon saw me walking the floor with Stephen again. I felt it would be awful to have to leave him while he was like this – not really well. At around three o'clock I felt the first real pains – not bad at all, but slightly more than twinges. After about ten minutes I decided to phone Rick's office but he still wasn't back from his meeting. The girl on the switch said she'd get him to phone as soon as he got back. Margaret called again and said to leave Stephen any time. The pains eased off again.

At around four o'clock I got Stephen off to sleep and put him up in the cot. Then Rick phoned and said he'd come home straight away. When he got back we hung around the house for the best part of an hour. The pains started again. On the rare occasions that Stephen took an afternoon nap it would be a very short one so I had suggested we wait until he woke up himself and then leave. But of course that afternoon, because we wanted him to wake up he had other ideas and with the heavy cold he slept deeply. By around half past five Rick could stand it no longer and decided to wake him and get me to the hospital. We left him down to Margaret's. I really felt a heel handing him over, my gorgeous baby who was off colour. He looked at me solemnly, and I felt as if he was berating me, or incredulous that I was actually going to leave him with the strings of his hat hanging down on either side of his face. Margaret wished me good luck.

The journey was easy for me – the pains had eased off again and I began hoping that they wouldn't send me home again. Once you've made the decision to go to the hospital you don't want to be told to go home again and wait. When we got there nervousness took over. We went upstairs with a nurse. Rick waited outside while I was sent into a little room and got undressed. The nurse examined me but seemed unsure whether or not anything was happening. She called the doctor who, luckily for me, was the one who had seen me before, the one who had referred me to the heart specialist. I was glad then that I'd had that man at the check-up on the Monday if it meant I got her for my labour. She told me I was two centimetres dilated. She said that meant the baby was saying: 'I'm here, I'm getting ready to come out.' However, given my dates, she said, she thought it would be best if I went on a drip for as long as forty-eight hours to try to stop the labour. She said they would give me two injections also, twelve hours apart, to develop the baby's lungs as, she explained, immature lungs were the biggest problem for premature babies. She said she would confer with a colleague but that probably he would agree that this was best.

My heart sank. Trying to turn the baby back. This scenario had never occurred to me. All I wanted to do was get the labour over with now that I'd started. I had not envisaged this at all and I was already tired from the lack of sleep the previous night.

I was brought into the labour ward and Rick was allowed in to see me so I was able to tell him what was happening. A short time later the doctor came back and confirmed that they were going ahead with the drip. I was also linked up to a machine which monitors the baby's heart. The nurse let me hear it, bumping away. That was reassuring but I was a bit apprehensive about the drip and didn't relish the thought of any chemical dripping into my bloodstream.

The doctor said I should be kept in the labour ward and also monitored carefully because of my heart murmur. When the drip was set up I had my first injection. Then Rick was allowed back in again. We chatted and tried to adjust to the new situation. The doctor had also told me the baby was small and that she would put the neonatal unit on standby to take the baby if it was born. I, for my part, had told her guiltily that I had changed my dates by one week but she didn't seem to think that made a great deal of difference. The baby was still about six weeks premature. She told us the baby would almost certainly have to go into an incubator. So now we had to face the prospect of the baby being taken away from us. However, we hoped that might only be for a week or so. All I knew was that I would be thrilled when it was all over.

They gradually turned up the drip and it certainly had uncomfortable side-effects – making my heart thump and head pound. It was a bit like running hard on concrete but without the option of stopping and letting my heart slow down again.

Rick and I wondered about work – my job – and whether I would be allowed back if they did succeed in stopping the labour. We decided I'd better ask the doctor about that.

When the drip became really uncomfortable the nurse turned it down again. She and the doctor later discussed my 'tolerance' of it. The nurse assiduously took my blood pressure and pulse.

The next time the doctor called up I was fairly well established on the drip. Rick was asked to leave again and she said she would do an internal examination – a less-than-enjoyable experience, to understate it, particularly when you are also hooked up to a drip, and tense.

Afterwards I asked her about work. She said we should certainly let them know that I would not be back in this week. 'You may not be back at all,' she told me. 'At least not until after you've walked out of here with a baby in your arms.'

She told me she knew it would be difficult to sleep on the labour ward but that I should try, and that I would be given the second injection early the next morning. She said it would be better if Rick went home as nothing was likely to happen during the night and, if it did, they would phone him.

After Rick and I had said our goodbyes I thought once more

of its being Denise's birthday and how strange that was and how the baby could well have been born that night if it had been let. Then I tried to sleep.

It was a very long night. Every time I seemed to drop off I would be woken by the screams, or moans, of a woman close to giving birth. Almost invariably this would be followed five or ten minutes later by the more distant sound of a newborn's first cries drifting down from the delivery room. I felt I'd given birth to about fifteen babies that night.

At one stage a poor woman was brought into the room I was in and she was terribly upset because, apparently, she'd screamed loud and long.

Added to the noise, I was still experiencing some discomfort from the drip. I couldn't turn over or move too much and every so often my blood pressure was still being taken.

I started to envy those women crying out in pain. I wished they'd let me experience it – let me go through it and have it all over, instead of trying to turn the baby back. I dreaded the thought of their succeeding and of having to go home and wait to go through it all again.

I was glad to see the dawn lighting the ward and I cried a little bit. Then a really kind young nurse came to help me wash, as I couldn't get out of bed and she brushed aside my apologies and said I shouldn't worry if I cried – that I was doing very well. She was really so encouraging.

My doctor was in very early – she'd been on duty all night. She gave me another internal examination and a short time later I was given my second injection to help the baby's lungs develop. At this stage I still felt quite bright and slightly refreshed from my few hours' sleep.

As I was now a fixture on the ward they decided to feed me. I was very hungry as I'd eaten nothing since lunchtime the day before. I especially enjoyed the cup of tea I was given for breakfast.

They were still adjusting the drip up and down every so often. Now there was a slight but growing difference in that every time they turned it down the pains were noticeable and when they turned it up the discomfort increased but the pains stopped. At least I was tolerating the discomfort better but I really felt I was between the devil and the deep blue sea.

The morning was long and slow but anything was better than the night and I was glad of the daylight bustle. Sometime before nine, two women came into my six-bedded room to be induced. All of the beds in each room have curtains around them, forming cubicles so I couldn't actually see anybody else, only hear them. One of the women was put in the cubicle right beside me, on my left. I could hear her chatting away to the nurse as she got ready for bed and had her drip set up. I envied her too and her certainty that it would all be over by that night.

I suppose the turn of events and all that had physically happened to me had forced my fears about this quiet baby to the back of my mind. They were still there somewhere though. The baby was certainly no more active, in spite of all that was going on, but I had to concentrate on the present, on getting through this day, so I couldn't afford to dwell on other, darker possibilities. I knew, too, that I was very tired. I didn't know how I would last another night and day on this drip and then, perhaps, after it all, go through a labour. I didn't feel confident about how I would handle it.

At some stage the sister called round and she told me someone had phoned for me – a neighbour, she said, who was minding my other child. It must have been Margaret. I wondered how Stephen was.

At around twelve Rick came. I was so glad to see him. It

17

seemed so long since the previous evening. He, of course, hadn't had a full night's sleep either. When he'd gone home he had called to Margaret and Don. They had already brought Stephen's cot down to their house and put him to bed there. Rick told me Stephen's cold was quite bad still but that he wasn't in too bad form. He said he'd wanted to spend some time with Stephen before leaving him down to the babyminder's.

We talked about my situation then. At one stage I laughed to think that I might have my baby before two other people I knew: one was the wife of my immediate boss at work. When I'd first told him I was pregnant again his reaction had been 'So long as it's not January, is it?' Because that was when his wife was due their second. Also, a girl at work expecting her third, but who was always overdue, had gone on maternity leave a couple of weeks previously but still hadn't had hers.

Rick said he'd go and get the paper and did I want anything. I said a magazine. It was a sunny, blustery day. I remember that part as being the best bit of the day – having Rick with me again, before exhaustion caught up with me and while the discomfort wasn't excessive.

My doctor came round and I was examined internally again. She was apologetic, but said that that was the most accurate way of assessing the situation. Still no one told me how long I would be on the drip. I was still working, with dread, on the basis of forty-eight hours.

The woman in the cubicle beside me was checked every so often. She was still cheerful but was getting pains. I never actually set eyes on her but she will always be part of that day.

After lunch my pains started to get just a bit stronger when the drip was on its lower level. It was nothing I couldn't manage but it was noticeable.

Then I began to feel myself starting to unravel. For no apparent reason my morale plummeted and I began to feel I wouldn't be able to go on going through all this for another twenty-four hours. The more I thought of the length of time ahead the more downcast I became.

A nurse came and told me that Mary from work had phoned and that she'd heard I'd already had the baby. The nurse said she'd told her no, that they were still trying to turn back the labour, but without much success.

When she'd gone I realised this was a chink of hope: that I wouldn't have to go through all this again, that I would at least have the baby in the next day or two.

My doctor came round again about three and I had yet another internal examination. The nurse had also told her that my pains were getting a bit stronger. I felt I was quite different from the relatively optimistic person I'd been that morning: I felt dishevelled, discouraged and worried. The doctor told me that every hour I kept that baby inside me was helping it. That did serve to concentrate my mind. It was also another chink of hope that it might all come to an end – if she was now talking in terms of hours rather than days.

Rick also managed to talk to her himself and when he came back he told me she'd said they always tried to balance the needs of the mother with the needs of the baby and that they wouldn't push me too far.

That long, long day dragged on. It got to the stage when the pains were seeping through, despite the drip. I told the nurse. The drip was not going to work. They couldn't turn this baby back.

At around five o'clock the sister told me they would be turning the drip off at about seven. I would have been on it for twenty four-hours by then. I was both relieved and nervous. I told her I was worried about how I'd cope with the labour as I was so tired. She said it would probably be fairly quick because the baby was small. She said they didn't want to give me pethidene because the baby was so premature. I said I hadn't needed it with Stephen, that I'd managed fine with the gas and air.

The pains were slowly getting worse, in spite of the drip, and for the last hour I found I was doing my breathing exercises, although also able to talk in between. Rick was with me, beside me. He was my security.

The time finally came to remove the drip and things did move quickly from then on. I was aware that the girl in the next cubicle was also in quite a lot of pain by now. I breathed as best I could and they brought me the gas in a while and Rick helped me with it. Being in labour seems to divide the mind from the body in some way, because while you're aware and able to think, your body has completely taken you over.

I was six centimetres dilated quite soon and I know by then I was starting to say to Rick 'I'm frightened' every few minutes. I don't know where the words came from or why I kept saying them: whether it was because I was so tired, just because of the labour, or because one bit of my mind, without ever putting it into words up to now, was desperately afraid that there might be something wrong with the baby.

I had only taken about three whiffs of gas when the nurse asked me if I'd any urge to push. I hadn't; but a couple of minutes later I had − a very strong urge. Next thing I was being speeded down the corridor to the delivery room. Rick was beside me again. I pushed. I pushed again. 'Your baby's head is born,' the sister said. There were two doctors there as well, a man and a woman. That was the last moment of our world as we knew it, that moment when our baby's head was born but not its body. One more push and the body came out.

The awfulness began.

The cord is very long. The cord's very long. They were almost shouting first. I leaned up to look at the baby, waiting for them to tell me whether it was a boy or a girl. When Stephen was born they had asked me which it was but I was so out of it they had had to tell me. This time I had been determined I would look and see for myself. All I saw was a huge red growth, seemingly out from the baby's stomach.

'There's a problem with your baby,' the male doctor said as he immediately began suctioning mucus away from it. 'Your baby's got a problem,' he repeated between sucks. Our baby cried then, a big, strong cry. There seemed to be nothing wrong with its lungs. In the near panic they decided to take it away and put a dressing on it.

So, already, one minute or less after birth, our baby was taken from us.

I kept asking the sister, 'Is it serious?' Insisting, staring into her eyes, as I lay, feeling totally helpless. She kept saying she didn't know, she really didn't know. I knew she did. But then I suppose I knew too.

None of this was normal but my reasoning seemed to have gone haywire and I couldn't think anything through myself. All the same I felt angry at not being told anything.

I was told more than enough soon enough. The panic left me then as what I was told was worse than anything I could ever have imagined. We were both catapulted into shock and grief. The information all seemed to come to me through the sister. My ears seemed tuned only to her voice. She'd got me through the birth. Now I heard only her.

'Your baby weighs about four and a half pounds.' But that wasn't an exact weight, she told me, because of the dressing. It was better than we'd been expecting. Four and a half pounds was not so bad. Babies are discharged from hospital once they reach five pounds. The next piece of information was less good: 'Your baby's going to have to go to Crumlin hospital. It's the best place for it.'

She said they would get on to them now and see if they could get a place as soon as possible. She said Crumlin was very busy so they might have to wait but that they would let us know. It was arranged that Rick would go down to the neonatal unit and wait to hear about Crumlin. Then the baby was brought to me to hold.

The third piece of information that stuck in my mind and is still stuck in my mind, and always will be, made my heart stop and the full impact of the situation start to hit home. The sister said: 'Your baby's in no immediate danger.'

It was serious. It was very serious. It was so serious our baby could die. Not tonight. Not immediately, but at some time in the future. Its future was uncertain.

The little thing was handed to me. It was my moment, the mother's moment, the moment the baby was almost mine and it was to be a long time before I felt that again. Wrapped in a green, hospital blanket, the little face was still and peaceful, the nose quite prominent in the face because it was thin. The baby felt light. I memorised the face as best I could, looked hard at it. As hands reached to take the baby away from me I quickly turned to Rick, wanting him to have the chance to cradle it too for a few moments. No one stopped me so he got his turn too.

They had to label the baby's wrist and ankle. The sister began writing, calling the words out to me, making me understand what I couldn't bear to hear. She called out my name, 'Mary Frances Boyle, 21 January, sex not determined.' Is that going to be a problem she asked, with family and friends and so on? Rick said no and I felt angry again at the ludicrousness of the conversation. I wanted to curse and scream at her: 'Of course it's a problem!' but nothing came out. Problem was too small a word for it. It was a disaster. It was terrible. No words could describe it. It was worse than anything I could ever have believed possible.

The label was put on the baby's ankle. The 424th birth in the hospital so far that year. The other label was put on the baby's wrist. The birth took place at 20.26 hours.

My life, our life together, would never be the same again. Everything was divided into before and after that moment.

The last question I was asked in the delivery room was whether we had picked a name for the baby. We hadn't. They asked us no more.

I was taken to the recovery room. Another nurse was with me. I felt sore now. I was in despair and exhausted. She put her arms around me and told me to cry, to let it out. I could only cry silently.

Rick was no longer with me. He must have been down in the neonatal unit. A woman was wheeled into the cubicle next to me. I heard her voice and knew it was the woman who'd been in the cubicle next to me all day, the one who'd been induced that morning. She had had a boy. She was tired but delighted, of course. She was chatting to the nurse with her. I so envied her. I felt I'd been through the mill too and now look where I was. It seemed so unfair. And the baby had been taken away. The baby with no sex.

The nurse decided I needed sedation. She wanted to give me something. I didn't want anything but she was quite insistent. In the end she agreed to give me only a half-dose of pethidene. Certainly I felt sore as I had had a very natural birth – no more than a couple of whiffs of gas and air. The pethidene, presumably, had some effect but did not immediately knock me out or seem to dull my perceptions. All I wanted now was to go home, to get up and leave this awful place but of course I wasn't going to be allowed do that.

Another woman was now in the cubicle opposite me. Her husband was comforting her. Then the chaplain came up to her. He told her they had baptised her baby but not to worry, that was just a precaution. I wondered vaguely what her problem was but was pretty well absorbed by my own situation. If only the baby was a girl, I thought, there would be some hope of simulating normality.

A nurse came to see me then, the same nurse I think. She told me they had baptised my baby in the unit and called it 'Frances'. She said they had seen that my second name was Frances and so had picked that. In fact Frances was not my second name at all but only my Confirmation name. When I had registered with the hospital on my first pregnancy the nurse had begged for a second name in case I'd be mixed up with anyone else so I had suggested my Confirmation name and she had eagerly typed that in so that it appeared on all my charts and labels and everything to do with me from then on.

It was ironic. I had never thought my Confirmation name could possibly be so useful. I felt deeply grateful to the nurse or doctor who had picked this unisex name for our baby. Now at least it had one of the labels essential in our society: a name. No sex, but a name. Francis, Frances, whichever it was to be.

Rick came back in to me. He had been down in the neonatal unit. He said the woman doctor who had been at the birth had said the baby was more than likely a boy, that boys were more likely to be born with these types of problems than girls. This was not what I wanted to hear. I said to Rick that I really hoped it was a girl. If it was a girl, I said, there was some hope, but if it was a boy there was none, it could never be normal. Huge presumptions on my part.

Much later it became clear that we had already diverged, Rick and I, that early, that soon after the baby's birth. He believed what the doctor had said to him and in his mind, from that remark onwards, thought of the baby as a boy. I wished intensely that the baby would turn out to be a girl and heard the boy supposition at second hand.

A nurse brought me a photo of the baby. It was a terrible photo and I didn't want it. It upset me again. I asked Rick to take it away, saying I would prefer to remember the baby as it was when we held it. Side-by-side with my desire to be told we had a girl was the knowledge that this baby might well die.

'No immediate danger' was branded into my brain. The imminent transfer to Crumlin was another factor. I was not absolutely certain that I would ever hold the baby again. Neither, had I asked myself then, was I at all sure I wanted it to live.

The chaplain came to see me briefly. I don't know what he said to me or I to him.

Rick said they had to wait until there was a bed free in Crumlin but that he would stay and go up there whenever the baby was transferred. We said our goodbyes and goodnights and he said he would phone my parents and Margaret and Don and leave the rest until the morning.

My heart went out to him. He would have to face that journey to Crumlin on his own. Also because he would have to break the news to people. So much already seemed to be falling on his shoulders while I lay in that bed, a very unwilling patient.

Rick took the photo home with him.

2

HOSPITAL

I was moved down to a ward. It was dark and quiet. The bed bumped up against the wall. For a few hours I slept – exhausted, and I suppose the pethidine helped. Around three o'clock in the morning there was some movement and noise which woke me. It was another woman being moved into the bed opposite me after having her baby.

Almost as soon as I woke the nightmare situation came back to me and I started crying again. I didn't think I was making any noise but the nurse must have heard me. She turned and asked me if I was crying. I said yes. The other nurse asked what was wrong and she told her I'd had a baby earlier in the night that had had to be taken to Crumlin.

After a while I dozed again, then woke, wishing the night was over and dreading the day to come. From the moment the baby was born I felt there was a huge weight over me, a dark shadow across my life. Every morning I woke to meet it to a greater or lesser degree. Sometimes it was like a broken heart, sometimes a gnawing worry, more often an angry resentment.

A very kind nurse came to bring me for my bath. The fact that our baby was not well, was not 'normal', made no difference to my body. My body was fresh from giving birth – sagging tummy muscles, swollen on top. I dreaded the milk coming to no purpose. The bath and facing my own body was one hurdle. Breakfast was the next.

With daylight I discovered that two of the women in my room were pre-natal and in for bed-rest. The third, the young woman who had arrived in the middle of the night, had had a baby boy. She was in the bed opposite me. It was her first and she was waiting to be transferred to a private room as soon as there was one free. The nurse who had given me my bath afterwards brought the baby down to her. She was, naturally, delighted. The nurse showed her how to clean him. One cotton wool ball for each eye, wipe outwards and so on, and how to change his nappy. It was purgatory to watch. I kept thinking that should be me too, I should have a baby too.

I sat down to breakfast with the two pre-natal women. I could feel the coming conversation. It was inescapable. It was to be the first of many. I wanted to run away and hide in a hole in the ground. As she put sugar on her cornflakes the more chatty of the two asked me if I had had my baby. Yes, last night, but it had to go to Crumlin.

'What did you have?'

The looming, obvious question we had no answer for.

'They don't know yet.'

I could see the blank look on her face, almost disbelief.

'I suppose it was so small they couldn't see,' she said, as if by way of explanation to herself. And tears dripped into my cornflakes.

Later in the morning the staff nurse came around and spoke to me, and said if there was anything at all they could do for me or anything I wanted, just to say. She told me the baby was in the Special Care unit in Crumlin and that myself and my husband could go up and visit later if we wanted.

I didn't particularly want to. I couldn't wait to get out of, and away from, the Coombe but I didn't particularly want to go to Crumlin.

The woman in the bed opposite me kept pretty much to herself but at about lunchtime her husband came in and they were admiring their new baby. If that woman only knew the torment she put me through that day when the last thing I wanted to see was someone else's perfect baby. It was a selfish but instinctive reaction.

The chaplain came to see me again. I felt sorry for him. He was young. What could he know about it all? What could he say to people like me. I was not in the humour for platitudes. He didn't offer me any. I said that if the baby could not lead anything like a normal life then I thought it would be better if it died. He didn't disagree with me. I respected him more for what he didn't say and could have. At the same time I felt that nothing and no one could alleviate my misery.

Later, the doctor who had looked after me so well all through the drip and labour, came up to see me, which I felt was very kind of her. She just came and sat on the side of my bed and said: 'I'm so sorry, so sorry. And after all you'd been through.'

I was doubly grateful to her for that. She had seen me go through it. She was giving me credit for my ordeal and for its end result. Nobody else did. I felt she really understood. She said I'd never forget that January.

Rick came in just after lunch. He had been in Crumlin until two o'clock in the morning. He said he had followed the ambulance from the Coombe up to Crumlin and that Francis had been in an incubator. Then he had been asked to wait outside the ward but he had sat there for nearly two hours and no one had come to him. Eventually he had knocked at the door and a nurse had come but the doctor had left by then. He said they'd forgotten that he was waiting outside.

Rick told me he didn't know if they could do much with Francis, that he had got the impression they might not be able to do much. Even then I began to realise I was half-hoping the baby would die. I felt ashamed of what my body had produced, of the terrible deformity that had been born out of me.

Rick said there had been snow on the car when he'd come out of Crumlin but that he had got home OK. I asked him had he phoned people and how had he managed. He had rung his Mum, who lives outside Manchester and that had been hardest of all, to tell her. He had also phoned Denise, my office and his office. I asked about Stephen. He said his cold was still bad but that just seeing him would have cheered me up.

Everyone presumed I was going up to Crumlin. I wasn't asked if I'd like to or if I felt up to it, in which case I probably would have said no. I was simply told I could. A nurse got me my clothes and pulled the curtains around my bed. Like an obedient child, knowing I ought to go, I got dressed. We set off in the car. I felt I had been away from the world for ages and even now was not quite part of it, as all the people and traffic around us were going about their normal Friday business. It had somehow become irrelevant to me. Yesterday seemed such a long time ago and today was suspended somewhere outside reality. I wasn't out in the real world anyway; I was just following a line from one hospital to another.

We got to Crumlin and Rick remembered the way up to the first floor. The Special Care unit was always called 'Special Care' or 'SCU' but when you go there first you see 'St. Patrick's' written over the door. We peeped through into a corridor and knocked on the glass. A nurse saw us and came out. We introduced ourselves as Francis Boyle's parents and we went into the first room on the left. To me, that day, it was horrific, awful. The baby was inside what looked like a huge machine, lying, strung out, blindfolded and very small, with a drip coming from somewhere and a nappy that looked too big for it.

Immediately I was both impressed by, and resentful of, the nurse. Her kindness, her gentleness, were immediately obvious. That impressed itself on me. It's hard to pinpoint my resentment, which was more complex. It was partly because of her real care – love if you want to call it that – for the baby in her charge, which I felt, even as its mother, I could not match. But it was also her presumption of our love and care for the baby, which I felt I could not live up to, that nearly made me feel I was there under false pretences. I did not love this baby. I did not care for it. It was mine but I didn't want to have to be responsible for it. I didn't want to take on the huge burden it represented for me, I didn't feel I could cope with its terrible deformities. I felt both guilty because I did not feel love for it and angry that it was presumed I would.

Ursula explained that Francis was under lights because he was jaundiced, which, she said, wasn't unusual for premature babies and that the blindfold was just to protect his eyes. She referred to the baby as 'he'. She said he was producing urine and dirtying nappies although, and this was the only time she faltered, she said they didn't know quite how it was coming out or where exactly. She peeped behind the nappy, opening one side of it, and we caught a glimpse of his lower body and the growth out from it.

Ursula asked me if I would like to hold the baby but I said no, especially as it was hooked up to so many things. She said he wasn't really, that he wasn't on anything apart from the lights and that it was just a saline drip. She told us he was sucking away on the soother. That was true: he was intermittently sucking on it and then it would fall out and roll down the big expanse of the huge incubator. It was an orange soother.

Someone got chairs for the two of us. We sat there, holding hands. Every time we faced something difficult together in the coming days and weeks and months we held hands. It literally gave me physical strength.

We sat and looked at our baby. I felt torn apart. I wanted the baby to die. Already I wanted it to die. I suppose I was still in shock and just wanted it to all go away as if it had never happened. My emotions were selfish but I couldn't help them. I felt I had produced a monster who didn't even have the basic prerequisite for living on this planet – a sex. Most of all I felt angry, angry that this had happened to me, to us. Why me? Why us? It wasn't fair.

The nurse's skilled hands would reach into the incubator and gently touch the tiny body and the baby would give little reflex jerks. The only other features I really noticed were its hands and feet and ears. They seemed huge in relation to the size of the body. The ears were long and pointed. They reminded me of a pixie's in a children's book. The feet were pointing noticeably up towards the head.

It was terribly warm in the room, like all hospitals. After a few minutes of sitting I could feel myself getting sleepy and an almost irresistible temptation to let my head drop down. I really had to fight to stay awake. The nurse asked me if I was all right. She said I looked pale, she was sure I must be exhausted. It was less than twenty-four hours since the birth.

We didn't stay all that long. She told us we could come any time to see Francis. We went out into the corridor and out through the heavy wooden doors of the ward onto the landing. We walked back down the wide wooden staircase, holding hands, and out to our car.

Rick drove me back to the hospital. My aunt and uncle had called while we'd been out and had left a card and note to say how sorry they were. I pulled the curtains round the bed, got undressed again and lay on my bed, exhausted. Rick said goodbye soon afterwards and set off for home and Stephen.

I felt sorry for myself. It was all so different from when Stephen was born, when it had all been cards and flowers and congratulations. This time round there were no congratulations and I felt I deserved them even more because I'd been through so much harder a time. On the other hand perhaps we don't deserve congratulations at all when we have a baby, I thought. After all, it's just good or bad luck whether you have a healthy one or not; it's nothing to do with how wonderful you are.

The hardest thing was having no baby to hold or show off or dress. I had no little crib beside my bed, nothing at all after all that.

It was soon visiting hour and the woman opposite me had a large group around her bed, congratulating her and admiring her little boy, asking her what it had been like and how she felt. All the normal conversations that are repeated hundreds of times a day around a maternity hospital. One of the relations said: 'Sure as long as it's healthy nothing else matters,' and I felt like screaming.

Soon afterwards a nurse came in and said there was a private room free. She helped the woman to pack up her things and wheeled the baby, in its cot, out of the door ahead of her. The relief when she was gone was enormous. It was nothing personal. I would have quite liked a room on my own, just to be able to cry in peace, but I knew I was better off to stay where there were people around me.

Teatime came. I felt hungry again. I even felt bad to feel hungry, as if that was another sign of not caring. I dreaded the 'blues' arriving in a couple of days' time, because already I felt as if I couldn't possibly feel much worse. I also dreaded getting the milk. I couldn't stop my body producing it. I couldn't tell my body it had made a terrible mistake by holding on to that baby. My body was outside my control. It knew it had produced a baby so it would also produce milk as day follows night.

I had planned to breastfeed but now felt it was out of the question. I suppose it was another form of rejection but it was also impractical. The baby was sick and it was not with me. I would practically have had to live in Crumlin to try it. Attempts at expressing milk when I'd been feeding Stephen had been spectacularly unsuccessful so I didn't think that was an option either. Anyway Stephen needed me too. After all, he was still only a baby himself and I didn't want to neglect him. Strangely enough, no one suggested breastfeeding to me anyway although I had expected them to mention it. No one, not even any of the nurses, asked me if I'd intended to feed the baby myself. I didn't bring it up either. Rightly or wrongly, I interpreted this as another sign of the seriousness of the baby's condition.

After tea I felt so bad I wondered what I could possibly do to cheer myself up, even a little bit. I decided to phone my sister, Denise, in London. I can pour my heart out to her in any difficulty without feeling self-indulgent because she will always listen and be as interested as I am. My brother-in-law, Ken, answered the phone.

'Well, Denise isn't actually here. At this moment she should be in Heathrow waiting to get on a plane to Dublin. She decided she had to come over and see you for the weekend.'

I was surprised and grateful to her. It certainly was the best thing she could have done for me – to bring herself.

Ken asked me how the baby was. I told him we'd been up to see it and didn't really know any more yet about how things stood. He said he was thinking of us and to give his love to Rick.

I wandered around the corridors and then lay on my bed again. There were only the husbands of the other two women in the ward for evening visiting hour. Pre-natal cases don't attract anything like the number of visitors that new mothers do. It was quiet. The next thing my father and mother were in the doorway.

My mother suffered from Parkinson's disease and was not at all well. My father helped her across the floor and, in his usual awkward way, got her a chair and half-helped, half-shoved her into it. My father was always like a bull in a china shop – awkward, funny, maddening, but always cheerful, big-hearted, full of ideas and eager to talk to everyone.

My mother sat very close to me and clasped my hand tightly. She was too exhausted from the journey into the hospital to speak just yet. But she had come. That was enough. I knew it was an enormous effort for her – an eight-mile car journey and then a short walk and stairs, particularly this late in the day when she was far from her best. Just her being there said how much she cared, cared deeply and was so sorry for me. Just seeing my mother set me off again, briefly, and I shed a few more tears.

My mother had had Parkinson's disease for almost as long as I could remember. I do recall her and my father at the tea-table one evening telling Denise and me that she had it. It sticks in my mind, like other moments from childhood, less because it meant an awful lot to me at the time but more because it was obviously of such major importance to them and that gravity was conveyed to me. The other fact that had filtered through and stuck was that the disease would get worse. It had.

Slowly, insidiously, over the years, my mother had deteriorated to the point where no drugs could control her symptoms for more than short, unpredictable periods of time. Now she had difficulty walking and speaking, and even doing the simplest things that most people take for granted, like swallowing or holding a mug of tea. It is a terrible disease and it had taken over her body.

My mother's life of illness, her seemingly endless deterioration, her brave and persistent efforts to retain her dignity against all the odds, and the years I had spent watching her had had a deep effect on me and on us as a family. Inevitably through my own childhood and adolescence I had been influenced by what I had to watch her suffer and by her own views on life and her situation in particular. In my own eyes it partially explains my attitude towards our baby although I don't say it excuses it.

My mother had often felt in the years prior to this that she would be better off dead: that her life was not worth living. She could do so little for herself. She could not drive a car, go out, mix with people. She could enjoy so little, sometimes not even small family gatherings, and felt at ease with very few people. She might be able to participate for an hour or so. More often than not the tremors got so bad that she could focus on nothing else and sometimes had to go and lie down. In recent years she had suffered from depression and become very withdrawn. She was like a hostage but with no hope of being released alive – her only hope of release was to die. It was always difficult to encourage her when she said she would be better off dead because there was no denying it. Oh, we made encouraging noises and spoke of how she had us to live for and my father, and now Stephen, but really we knew that if we were her we would often wish to be dead ourselves.

That evening, as she sat beside me, upset for me, I was not at all surprised when after a while she managed to say: 'It would be better for him if he didn't live, wouldn't it?'

I know she felt deeply for this, her second grandchild and I know she wanted what was best for him, the poor little thing. No one had more of a right to say that than her. I agreed with her but I felt it was, at least partly, out of my own selfishness rather than for any altruistic desire for what was best for the baby. I still wanted the situation to disappear and get back to where I'd been before all this, to escape. I wanted it all to be over, for someone to tell me it had just been a bad dream.

My father told me how he'd been just about to leave the house when my mother had said she'd like to come with him. I could just picture the scene. Probably my mother had been working up to that all day and to the effort it would entail. He said he'd been taken aback but had got her coat and got her into the car.

They didn't stay terribly long. My mother started to 'go off' as she called it, the phenomenon when the *el-dopa* drugs she was on started to wear off. She started to shake badly and my father decided to take her home. He led her out, holding her hand gallantly.

To think that I had once glibly said to Denise that all our children were bound to be healthy because of our mother's illness – that that was the ill-health in our family. On top of that I was a coeliac, which means I can't tolerate wheat and some other grains. I had been confident that that was our quota, that God couldn't possibly load any more onto us, so I had believed that her illness was nearly like an insurance policy against more, or worse. By all the statistics, I felt, any children we had should be healthy, that we couldn't be doubly unlucky. I'd been wrong.

Like ninety-five per cent of people in the Republic of Ireland I had been brought up a Catholic. My faith in a God was both firm and shaky. I could pray, and often did, to a childhood God, asking favours or blessings. From an adult, and more philosophical point of view, I found it all more complex, less clear-cut. The suffering that human beings experience on this earth I found, and still find, incomprehensible in the face of any benevolent God. Suffering may bring people closer together; good may come of it, I'm not denying that, but how any all-seeing, all-caring being could endure watching it, century after century, million after million, without intervening, yet remaining closely involved and deeply, personally loving each of those human beings, is beyond my comprehension.

How could he/she supervise carnage, ill-health, brutality, deformity, mental disability, how could he/she plan such a world for those he/she is supposed to care most about and use it as a way to test us and make us earn a place in a better existence? I thought about the whole problem a great deal in those early days. I had thought about it before, five years previously in particular, when my mother had been gravely ill and had suffered certain psychoses. I had worn myself out thinking about it then and in the end the single crumb of explanation that had made any sense to me was that perhaps in all my questioning and doubting I was closer to what I was seeking than when I was complacent and life was just ticking over. That still left my mother and her intense suffering unexplained.

Our baby was twenty-four hours old. I felt my life, our life, was over. I felt cheated of happiness, the happy years Rick and I might have shared. I felt angry at how hard God was making everything for us. I felt so sad for Stephen and what all this would do to him, how he would be cheated of the attention he deserved and saddled with a little brother with major disabilities. I felt for Rick too. I felt for him so much it hurt. I was appalled at what had befallen and I felt, I knew, I was partly to blame. I wondered if I had done anything to cause the deformities. Those thoughts still come back to haunt me sometimes. I wondered if Rick would have been better never to have met me.

Like all hospitals, the Coombe is awake and on the go early. We got the six-thirty cups of tea but, because there were no babies in our room, it stayed quiet for longer and we all lay in bed, dozing. Breakfast that morning was a lot easier than the first. These people knew now. I didn't have to explain myself again. One more day and I should be released.

I didn't want visitors and that was most unlike me. I'm normally a very sociable person and love having people around me. I couldn't remember feeling like that before – meeting people was so hard and for months that persisted. For once I couldn't splash my troubles around and so dissipate them. This time I felt cut to the quick.

At some stage that morning the staff nurse came down and sat on my bed and chatted to me. She told me the baby had had a stable night and that we could go up to visit again in the afternoon. She said we should try to visit as much as we could, especially if the long-term outlook wasn't too good. It was like an echo of the labour-ward sister's 'Your baby's in no immediate danger'. What they really seemed to be saying was that our baby was in danger, but not now, not yet. The nurse also said that if there was anything, anything at all that any of them could do for me I had only to ask.

Later that morning a close friend phoned me – another Mary. I was allowed to take the call by the nurses' station. Mary is always cheerful, always a tonic no matter how low your spirits are. That day I felt she was calling from very far away but I still felt touched by her going to the trouble to try and reach me in my 'prison', the hospital. She said she was thinking of me and to keep up heart and give her love to Rick. I was really grateful to her and glad to have talked to her. It was one of the nice things that morning.

The other was the arrival of Denise. She is always a tonic as well. No matter how bleak our predicaments we can share them and almost always have a laugh. We understand each other. Denise came mid-morning and hugged me, with tears in her eyes, and said how sorry she was. Then we both had a few tears but in the next moment she was presenting me with a bunch of flowers and a ridiculously small plastic vase that not a single stem would fit in, which made us both laugh.

She said she thought I should have flowers because after all I'd had a baby even if it was premature and had problems. She had exactly the right mixture of sympathy, celebration, realism and humour. She always has, for other people, while being far more critical and less objective about herself and her own achievements. She is one of the most generous people I've ever met – generous in giving of herself. We chatted about the baby, the possibilities, me. With Denise I didn't feel guilty talking about me, my feelings, my reactions.

Rick came in after an hour or so and again the curtains were pulled round my bed and I got dressed, like an obedient little girl. So ingrained seems to be my adherence to socially-acceptable behaviour that I wouldn't have dreamed of shocking, hurting and inconveniencing everyone by saying: 'No. I will not go. I don't want to. I can't face it.' Meekly I went with them.

Again the room in Special Care was a shock. In fact it was worse. A very ill-looking boy of six or eight was in a bed at right angles to our baby's incubator. His parents were there with him. The boy seemed to be unconscious and the nurse's comments less than optimistic. Chairs were brought for us and we sat down. The same nurse was looking after Francis. This time she opened the incubator, took off the black patches over the eyes, which she explained again were to protect them from the ultra-violet light rays. Gently, and skilfully, she wrapped a blanket around the tiny body and handed the baby to me to hold.

So, for the second time since the birth, I held my second child. Frances was tiny, so tiny and fragile. We each took a turn holding. Rick after me and then Denise. She was the most voluble by far of the three of us and kept exclaiming on how floppy his head was, just because he was premature. The nurse asked me how I was feeling and said how exhausted I must have been the day before. Rick, being the father, was not ever asked how he was. Then, gently, Frances was put back under the lights.

The mother of the boy came over to us and said she'd pray for us and she gave us a medal for Francis. I felt repelled by this, while realising she meant well. I had no faith in the medal to change this baby or situation.

Rick and Denise left me back at the Coombe. I had a few hours to put in. Denise had brought me a magazine as well but all of the topics seemed so ridiculously trivial and irrelevant that I could only glance through it. I dragged my way through the afternoon and tea. One of the women in the room had been allowed to go home. The other one was upset because she hadn't been discharged. I had technically been discharged but had to wait until the following morning to be allowed out. We didn't make the most cheerful of company for each other. I was relieved at least that there were no more babies in our room.

After tea one of the nurses came and told us we were moving as there was a woman on her own next door and they thought we'd be better off together. So we moved. This time, instead of the middle bed, I was put at the window, facing the opposite way. There was a woman in the bed across from me. We got talking, naturally. She told me she had had a stillborn baby on Thursday night – a little girl. It turned out to have been about fifteen minutes before I had had my baby. I thought what an awful night the labour ward must have been having – one stillborn baby and two sick babies all in one half hour.

There were now four of us in the room because there was also a very young woman who had been admitted with a threatened miscarriage that afternoon and was being kept in for observation. I cannot remember any of their names, only the story of the woman opposite me. She already had a son and a daughter in their teens and this pregnancy had been unexpected, I gathered, but not unwelcome. For two weeks before the birth this woman had known her baby was dead but she said she had looked perfect when she was born and they didn't know what had caused the death. They had been terribly nice to her, she said, and she'd been in a room on her own for the labour and birth. She had held the baby and it was now over in the morgue. They had told her she could go and see it again there but she said she didn't think she wanted to. They were going to bury her in the Holy Angels plot in Glasnevin. She said she'd been told to rest but that when she got home she knew she would start doing things. You have to do your bits and pieces, sure, don't you?, she said.

I'd briefly told her my position, about the baby, and Stephen at home, but, God forgive me, I envied that woman that evening. What wouldn't I have given to have had a stillborn baby. Then my suffering would be over and I would be starting the 'getting over'. I felt so miserable at the thought of what was ahead of me, us. It was all still too awful to take in completely. Of course, hand-in-hand with the feeling that I'd prefer if my baby had been stillborn, came the guilt for feeling that. And that was a cycle to be repeated, hundreds and thousands of times in the coming months.

The woman's family came in then, her husband and teenage children. You could see what a lovely family they were and their different relationships. The baby would certainly have been a very

41

exciting addition to the family. They had all spent months looking forward to, anticipating this little baby – nine months can be such a long, long time. And now there was no baby to bring home, just the emptiness of an unfulfilled promise. The children, I thought, would get over it, while never forgetting completely. The husband, too, I thought, would slip back into normality. Only the wife would be left at home with empty arms although she would resume her routines, carry on gradually and, as she said herself, start with her 'bits and pieces'.

My father and Denise came in to see me and the other two women's husbands arrived at the same time. My father chatted on about Stephen, who was the apple of his eye, although he still didn't sound well to me. I couldn't wait to get home and see him. The picture of him as I'd said goodbye three days ago, with his little hat and penguin suit, was like a snapshot in my mind, his little face solemn and staring, not quite fully awake. He was only a baby too and I needed him.

My father also said how amazing my mother had been to get in to see me. Only brief references were made to the baby. My father was always so deeply affected by the suffering of those close to him that he could hardly bear to think or talk about it. His suffering on our behalf and his sadness about the baby were things I hardly took account of in all those months ahead. I really feel that I should have noticed them more. But I was so utterly concentrated on getting through each day and so consumed by my own misery that, apart from Rick, I'd say I made little effort to be a comfort to anyone else.

Rick's mother was in the same position – hurting for both Rick and me as well as coming to terms with her sick grandchild. She's often said that when Rick rang her that morning with the news she so wanted to catch the next plane over just to be with us.

Denise had acted on a similar impulse, knowing that even long phone calls are no substitute for the real person or for a hug.

Denise said she'd be in with Rick the next morning to collect me and bring me home. We'd go up to Crumlin on the way and then out home. She asked me what clothes she should bring in to me. I picked the same skirt as when I'd been going home with Stephen. After all, that was less than eleven months previously. I didn't really care what I wore except that I didn't want to wear the clothes I had had on coming in. I never wanted to see those clothes again. I wanted to wipe out the whole pregnancy, forget it.

Although I kept thinking how desperately I wanted to get out of the hospital, the talk of clothes and going home made me realise just how much I had to face outside. The hospital was like a retreat house by comparison. I was in an insulated little world of nurses and patients. The only people I'd spoken to other than them were my immediate family and Mary on the phone. I wasn't at all sure how I was going to manage.

After the visitors had all gone we turned on the television. The girl with the threatened miscarriage had to stay in bed but the rest of us got up and sat around it on chairs. It was dark outside.

I thought how it was Saturday night – other people would be going out for a drink, going into town, going about their normal lives and here were we, all locked in our separate little miseries which none of us would probably ever forget. The *Late Late Show* came on. It was all I could do to watch it. Like the magazine it seemed so removed from my situation and so trivial.

A nurse came into the room. I looked up. It was the sister from the labour ward who had delivered my baby. If I'd been asked whether I would recognise her again if I'd met her on the street I honestly couldn't have said I would, but as soon as I saw her face and penetrating gaze I knew her so definitely I was back to Thursday night again.

She said I was looking a lot better than the other night. She asked me how I was and how the baby was. In Crumlin. In Special Care.

She said they'd been very busy. That this was the first night it had been quieter.

I'll always remember that sister for coming down to see me. I'll never know her name but she was there at the moment when the baby was born. When everything suddenly went wrong.

I was dying to get out of that hospital. I just could not wait. Still, I had to get through the routine. The breakfast, the chatter, the offer of Panadol. The woman opposite me decided, after all, to go down to the morgue to see her baby again. The girl in for observation had to stay in bed. Eventually, after what seemed like days more, Denise and Rick arrived. They pulled the curtains round my bed and I got dressed. I said goodbye to the others in my room and to a couple of nurses. Then I walked down the flight of stairs to the front entrance.

I had a tight, painful feeling inside me: this should have been so different. I should have been walking down these stairs with a nurse carrying my baby. Instead I was leaving without any baby. There should have been the ceremony of taking off the baby's identification tags, off the arm and ankle with me, the proud mother, acknowledging that this was my baby, born on 21 January at 20.26 hours. Then the nurse would put the baby into the car and we would drive away. We were walking down the stairs without any nurse and I felt it was so unfair and I was selfish to be thinking only of myself and how unfair it was.

We went up to Crumlin. The older child was still in the same room and seemed unconscious. The parents weren't there and I was glad. Again nurse got chairs for the three of us and we sat around the incubator. The baby's nappy was open and we could see all of the baby's body, in all its abnormality. The nurse was kindness itself, asking me how I felt and again saying how exhausted I must be. I used to feel bad for Rick because I seemed to be given so much attention and he so little. There were times when I felt like introducing him and pointing out: 'This is the father'. The nurse again let us hold the baby for a few minutes each. I found this upsetting and I was keyed up still, waiting for her to mention the ears and feet and tell us what was wrong with them. She deftly put the baby back into the incubator when 'our time was up'. Of course she didn't say that and of course the baby had to go back in but it was only with her agreement that we could hold the baby. That was one of the unavoidable, but hardest, things about hospital life: that we had no rights, ultimately. Everything you wanted to do you had to get permission for first.

That morning I felt angry and self-pitying. I still didn't particularly want to hold the baby but felt I was given little choice and it would have seemed so awful to refuse. But I despised myself for not having the guts to say no. I still didn't want this to be my baby. I felt no love for it. I wished it would die.

I keep saying 'the baby'. We did refer to 'Francis' quite a lot. That was a convenient tag and I was very grateful for the name many times in the next couple of weeks. But there was an enormous problem with pronouns. 'It' sounded so awful for describing a new baby and we avoided it. 'He' and 'she' were out of the question because neither applied, so we circumvented wherever possible, by referring to 'the baby'.

Once again that morning the heat and sitting down got to me and I began to feel uncontrollably drowsy, to my further shame.

The nurse suggested we might like to see the house doctor on

45

duty and we agreed. He was a tall, thin man, quite shy I would say, and certainly not a good communicator. He stood awkwardly by the incubator and spoke to the three of us without even first enquiring who Denise was. He told us the baby would need a number of operations. He said it was usually more successful if babies such as these were brought up as girls, even if they were boys. He left us in a state of shock.

This was a new, undreamt of horror, making everything else fade into insignificance. From that moment my longings that it be a girl were redoubled. I hoped beyond hope: 'If only it can be a girl . . . Please let it be a girl.'

Afterwards the nurse said the consultant would like to see us and could we come in to the hospital at half past eight the next morning? We said we could, again agreeing without question to something that would be difficult enough to achieve – getting across to Crumlin that early in the morning, with Stephen not so well.

Rick drove us home. Denise, as always, had a cheering effect on us but even she was shocked by the idea of having to bring up the baby as a girl if it really was a boy.

I had been really longing to see Stephen. It was the one thing I had been looking forward to. However, when we got to our house, I suddenly felt everything was unbearable. I got out of the car and stood looking at our house, crying bitterly.

It was only four days since I had walked out of that front door in some trepidation admittedly but basically full of hope. Now I felt our lives were ruined. I felt Stephen's life was going to be damaged terribly and the awfulness of our situation, compared with that short time ago, just hit me when I saw the front of our house. Instead of bringing a baby home I was bringing an enormous, invisible burden.

Rick comforted me, being strong, yet again, for both of us and we went in. When I'd calmed down, felt the strangeness and familiarity of being home, he asked me if I wanted to come down with him to collect Stephen. I did. I wanted to see Margaret and Don too, after all they'd done for us by looking after our other baby.

Stephen was crying when we arrived. Apparently he'd just banged his head. I felt he looked very different from when I'd left him and all my anxiety about him seemed to come to a head. There were a few ounces of milk left in a bottle and Margaret gave it to me. He sat up on my lap and slowly finished it off. Margaret said he'd refused to drink it for them. It was the right thing to say. For the first time in days I felt I was a mother again and I had a baby to hold and cuddle. That was one of the benefits of there being so little between the two: we did at least have another baby at home, a real baby, not a toddler or a little boy but another baby who couldn't yet walk or talk and who still needed bottles.

We drank coffee and talked a bit. Margaret had, at our request, found out about the legal position regarding us, the baby and treatment. She said that basically we had no rights: the hospital and doctors could decide what to do and how to treat our baby. I felt I wanted as little intervention as possible. The problems were so huge and so impossible to rectify that I felt nature should be allowed to take its course.

I thought of years ago when it wouldn't have been possible to treat Francis at all. It would have been a matter of keeping the baby comfortable and letting the little thing drift away peacefully. I thought of third-world countries, too, where the resources just wouldn't be there to care for our baby and it would die. I felt angry that we were caught in this situation where the very medical resources that could save so many lives were going to contrive to keep this, our baby, an aberration of nature, alive. I thought of third-world babies, born healthy and perfectly formed, who died simply from lack of food, and of all the money and technology being used to keep our very abnormal child alive so that he/she could lead a very abnormal life. I felt something was terribly wrong with the world and this was one dilemma that I never resolved while our child was alive and that still strikes me from time to time. In the end the only way I could rationalise it was by arguing that I happened to be born in this country, to this system, and therefore I had to accept what was done here. I had to accept the medicine on offer here and accept it on behalf of my child. However, these arguments were a long way down the road and at that stage, that Sunday, sitting in Margaret's front room they were at most half-formulated, half-registered in my mind. The dominant feeling when told about the abstract legal position was one of impotence again: we had no rights regarding our child and no say in what would happen.

Margaret stressed that her adviser had said the legal position would rarely, if ever, be followed to the letter. She said the hospitals and doctors would always consult the parents and try to agree on a course of action with them. But still, knowing how I felt and how my feelings would almost certainly be unacceptable in such a Catholic country, I found that of little comfort.

When we'd brought Stephen home my anxiety was such that I insisted Rick call the doctor even though it was Sunday afternoon. I said he wasn't well, that he'd had this dose now for four days and he could well need antibiotics. The doctor came fairly quickly. Rick ran out to him to warn him about our situation. That was one of the moments when I realised just how much stress he was under too. Although he was being so strong and seemed so calm outwardly he was, if anything, doing too much, rushing to attend to things, answer the phone and protect me. He seemed to be on overdrive. He was suffering terribly too. It was several years later that someone told us how difficult it is for couples to support each other in times like that. She said each partner is going through so much that it's almost impossible for them to also act as each other's chief support. If possible it's better to have someone else you can lean on also. But when you're going through it you just muddle on.

The doctor came in and commented: 'So you've been having a hard time.' He took Stephen's temperature and said he was sick, he was running a temperature but that he'd advise leaving him for another forty-eight hours to see if he could get over it himself before he'd prescribe antibiotics.

I don't remember much else about the day except that I felt completely exhausted and did very little. We went to bed very early, especially as we'd to be up to get to Crumlin for 8.30 am. Denise said she'd mind Stephen while we were there.

Stephen woke in the early hours of the morning. Denise got up with him. He was crying bitterly. Rick went to check that Denise was managing all right. I lay in bed feeling really strange. Here I was, in my own house, letting someone else look after my sick child. Admittedly it was my own sister, but still . . . At the same time I felt incapable of getting up myself.

In the morning it turned out Denise had sat up with Stephen for nearly three hours. That was probably the longest anyone had had to be up with him during the night since he was born. Probably, she said, she could have put him back in his cot, but she'd been afraid to in case she'd only disturb him again.

3

CONSULTATIONS

We were tense as we drove to Crumlin that morning. It was a grey, January morning, without much light. It seemed so long since Francis had been born and yet here we were, about to meet the surgeon in charge of the case for the first time.

He greeted us, shook our hands, commented that I looked very well considering when the baby was born. He couldn't remember exactly. Thursday evening, we told him. We were shown into a small room with one window. The surgeon sat over in one corner. We stood with our backs to the door. He paused and then he said: 'Your baby's condition is very rare and very severe.' Most surgeons such as himself, he said, would only come across one or two babies such as ours in their entire careers. He said it would require a great deal of surgery but that two major operations would be needed initially: one to separate out the bowel, involving a colostomy. The second operation, he said, would basically be to try and close the bladder. He estimated that there would be roughly a fifty-fifty chance in each case.

He said some of the intestine might be used for the second operation but that, very often in cases such as these the babies had a shorter than normal intestine and so there might not be enough to cut out any more.

Asked about the baby's sex, he said these types of problems tended to occur mostly in boys. But, he said, it had been found that given the type of problem it was almost always better to bring them up as girls. He said that would involve hormone treatment, and so on, but that, as girls, these children tended to be better-adjusted.

Our minds reeled. This confirmed what the house doctor had told us the previous day. Rick said our main priority was that Francis should not suffer more than was necessary. I asked whether the baby had to be operated on at all or could we decide it would be better if it weren't treated. In the scenario the professor had just outlined my wish for non-intervention was stronger than ever. I really wanted this baby of ours to die.

The surgeon thought about what I'd said. He never spoke without thinking out what he was going to say. He was obviously well used to dealing with parents, hundreds of them every year. He measured what he said carefully. Eventually he said that it was very difficult for him as a surgeon and that then there were the nurses to think of. He said it would be asking a lot of the nurses to care for a baby on that basis. And, he said, he'd have to consult with the chaplain to see what the ethics of the situation were.

He questioned our position, also. 'We would have to feed the baby,' he said.

We agreed. 'Of course, yes.'

We would have to continue treating the jaundice too, he told us, adding that untreated jaundice could cause brain damage.

Neither of us had realised this but we readily agreed to this too.

And then, he posited aloud, we would have to consider the situation should there be an infection: whether to treat it with antibiotics or to withhold them.

He left it at that but there was plenty for us to consider, as well. The implications of our position were certainly more complex than I had thought.

The situation was left like that. He said he would meet us again to discuss it further.

Once again we were in shock. That morning, although not as bad as the morning of the birth, certainly was one of the worst we had to experience. The horrific vista ahead seemed unbearable: to bring a child up as a girl knowing every day of its life that you were acting out a lie seemed something no one had a right to ask of us. Again, one wonders what, had it been carried to the ultimate, would the legal situation have been? Could we have been forced to do that against our wishes? From the coming days I realised just how persuasive the medical profession could be and how limited one's choices really were but I still baulk at the thought of what we were being asked to do. And beyond that loomed all the practical difficulties it would entail – the abnormality compounded by a living lie, the hormones – and would these ever be explained to the child? And what if she discovered she was really a he and wanted to change back?

I felt that the consultant that morning and at subsequent meetings did not fully realise how enormous the sexual aspect of the problem was to us. I did take in all he said about the operations, the bowel, the bladder and so on, but, being purely physical defects, they seemed of minor importance compared with the fundamental problem of what sex our baby was and what sex our baby was going to be allowed to be.

We went up to see our baby. Different nurses were on duty now that the weekend was over. You half-expected, although of course on thinking about it it didn't make sense, to see the same nurse every day. Now it was Monday. A new shift. More nurses to get to know. It was the very, very beginning of all we had to get to know, the hospital routine.

The nurses, without exception, were warm, skilled and caring women. I felt humbled by the love, and there is no other word for it, with which they treated our baby. Also, the respect. From day one that baby was an individual, a little person, in their care. They always spoke about their charge by name and described how things were going. They were totally different from the doctors. It was not only that they had different jobs. It was more than that. Their attitude to the 'patients' was also very different. Whereas the house doctors and surgeons, on the whole, seemed to see just that: a 'patient', a body that needed repairing or treatment, the nurses saw a person who needed care and love as well as treatment. They also spoke different languages. Granted, the nurses on the whole did not have to impart really bad news or take the decisions about treatment, operations and so on. They spoke a human language that you could relate to. The doctors tended merely to impart information and that sparingly. We needed so much more than just information.

Francis was still in the large incubator, like a table at a slant with a huge hood over it. He was still being treated for jaundice and indeed looked more golden now than at the beginning.

Francis, we were told, was doing fine, still producing bladder and bowel movements although they still weren't certain how and the jaundice, we were told, was very common in premature babies and should clear up.

We went home feeling worse than ever. Both of us found it awfully hard to come to terms with the idea of bringing our child up as the opposite sex to that with which he/she was born. It went against our instincts, somehow; it seemed an intervention beyond what was morally right and raised far more questions than it answered.

I kept saying I hoped Francis was a girl. Rick had been convinced by the doctor in the baby unit in the Coombe that Francis was a boy. The professor's supposition had confirmed this. For me, the consultant had merely stacked the odds against a girl but it was still a very open question and could go either way. So I went on hoping.

Stephen was still absorbing all our attention at home. He was still listless, with dulled eyes and hot hands, and I was frantic about him. I was afraid I was never going to get back the cheerful, healthy baby I had left when I was going into hospital and to some extent I was transferring my anxiety about Francis on to Stephen because his was a more tangible sickness. At one stage Denise even said to me, 'Well, Stephen isn't going to die, you know.' And that brought me to my senses because I realised I had actually been worrying that he might. I know that sounds crazy now, especially as the doctor hadn't even thought him bad enough to prescribe antibiotics but I had visions of pneumonia setting in and hospitalisation and eventualities which were out of all proportion to the situation.

Denise was, as always, her sympathetic self. She would look sadly at me and say something like, 'Well, the poor little fellow. He's sweet and at the moment all you can see is that he's very small and premature but you'd wonder all right what's best to happen and you're just going to have to see what does happen from day to day.'

Denise had to go back to London that evening so Rick took her to the airport. Again we went to bed very early, exhausted. That tiredness was so deep, I'll never forget it. It went on for weeks and weeks and it wasn't just me getting over the birth, although I suppose there was an element of that. It was more that we were both feeling a chronic tiredness. By half past eight or nine o'clock in the evening we were fit only for bed. I'm a wonderful sleeper and can sleep any time, anywhere, so I was not suffering from insomnia but I could never get enough sleep. I think it was a combination of shock and the constant using-up of nervous energy in those first few weeks that accounted for it. Certainly it seemed strange when people phoned to be told they'd disturbed us in bed before the main evening news was even over!

The following day, Tuesday, when we went in to Special Care Francis was no longer there but had been moved to Holy Angels, a baby ward. It was there that we first met Sr Anna. I immediately, and irrationally, resented her because, as I saw it, here was a nun who would take the Church line and who would certainly not share any of my more extreme views about the situation. Just then I didn't want anyone religious around me. I was in too much turmoil and felt no one could possibly understand what I was feeling or going through. I could not, with regard to Sr Anna, have been more wrong.

Seeing Francis in Holy Angels did give me a fright, however. In making this move the hospital seemed to be respecting our wishes. The ward was a long, narrow corridor of little individual rooms divided by wood and glass partitions. So a nurse with one baby in one cubicle could also see the babies on either side. Francis was still being treated for jaundice and was blindfolded. I was struck momentarily by the responsibility I would be taking on if I asked for our baby not to be treated but it did not in any way shake my resolve.

Sr Anna showed us into the room and spoke to us briefly. She also said the consultant would like to see us again the following morning at nine o'clock and was that all right? We said it was, once again knowing it would be difficult for us to get over to the hospital by nine. Poor Stephen, himself sick, was already being pushed around, I felt, at the expense of this, our second baby, who needed so much. My mind continued to go round and round, looking ahead, wondering how we could possibly cope, feeling it was so unfair on us, on Stephen. I felt God had no mercy. I felt no one who supposedly loved me could possibly do this to me, to us. Later I wondered how anyone who supposedly loved and created this baby could allow it to be born like this, so imperfect, so handicapped, so unsuited to a tough world.

At home I suggested to Rick that he should go back to work, that he could go in after we'd seen the consultant the following morning. He seemed reluctant and unsure. It was unlike him. He said things like: 'They understand. I've told them the situation.' And 'Well, if ever I needed time it's now. It's not as if I just take time off for any old thing.' He made no commitment as to when he would go back to the office.

Margaret agreed to look after Stephen from very early the next morning. I left him again with a heavy heart. Together Rick and I drove to Crumlin. Holding hands we walked up through the small hospital car-park, in the front door and up to the second floor. We pushed open the heavy wooden doors into Holy Angels and told a nurse we had an appointment. Sr Anna came to us and asked if it was all right if she sat in on the discussion. It wasn't really. I didn't particularly want her there but I was too polite to tell her so and so she showed us into an empty room.

The consultant had obviously thought carefully about what we had said and about our attitude generally. In the intervening forty-eight hours he had, true to his word, consulted various people. He had his position clearly thought out.

He told us he had consulted with the chaplain and that, in principle, they had no objection to not operating on Francis. He told us official church policy was that you should not use 'extraordinary means' to preserve life. That phrase recurred to me many times during the following months. I often wondered how exactly the church would define 'extraordinary means'. In a world of highly-sophisticated medical technology where exactly, I often speculated, would 'extraordinary' begin or end?

He told us he had also consulted with the nursing staff. Here he seemed to baulk a little. We were told again that it was asking a lot of them. He repeated that they would have to feed the baby, to treat the jaundice.

We agreed.

He said that, as we could see, they had transferred the baby to Holy Angels.

So far so good. But I felt they might simply have been testing our resolve. I didn't really think that we would be allowed to sit by and not let anyone near the baby.

Yes, the real issues were only just starting to emerge.

I said that what I really wished was that I could take the baby home and look after it there, simply feeding and caring for it like any other.

The consultant was visibly taken aback by this.

He made it clear that in his view this was completely out of the question. He asked us if we had seen all of the affected area. We said we had. Though the baby's problems were severe, he went on, we had to be clear that there was one major factor here for consideration in the equation and that was that we were dealing with intelligence. This seemed a key element for him. It was not something I had hitherto considered in any detail. I had, I suppose, taken it for granted that our baby had normal intelligence, that the problems were confined to the physical. It was certainly a forceful consideration but one which I needed to think through further.

He also told us that very often babies with problems similar to ours would have some other major problem such as a defective heart. In our case, however, everything else seemed to be normal.

That was the second serious factor in favour of intervention. He seemed to believe that the least we could do was to give our baby a chance.

However, he also had cogent points to put for the other side of the coin. He told us that, once the path of intervention was taken, it could be very hard for the baby to die. Given the sophisticated machinery at the disposal of the hospital, given the techniques available, life could be sustained, he said, against very many odds. All the same, he said, life could not be preserved against all odds and beyond a certain point things would take their own course but, he repeated, it could be very hard to die.

He said we had to make a decision: it was difficult, but by delaying they could be losing time. He said that by postponing surgery we could be making things more difficult to rectify. He didn't know for certain that that was the case, he stressed, but it was certainly possible.

His final statement was, for me, devastating: he told us we needn't think that by leaving our baby alone it would die. This wasn't necessarily the case, he said; it might well thrive; they simply didn't know. But, he said, if that were so and we later changed our view and opted for surgery then they might have lost precious time and it might be less successful.

What parent could resist such obvious logic? I felt we were being told that if we did not allow staff to intervene, then our baby's plight could be far worse. I felt the consultant's preference was for intervention but that he too had reservations. He seemed to recognise our dilemma and be sympathetic to our position. On the other hand, he had to think first of what was best for this baby. How could we, in our turn, refuse to take the path that might improve the baby's chances when not intervening could lead to even worse prospects?

His last statement, that we needn't think our baby would die if it didn't have surgery, hit me like an accusation: that I wished my own baby would die. That was true. I knew in my heart it was true. I just wanted the whole nightmare to go away. But I had been brought up to 'do the right thing', to obey authority figures, to comply. It was almost impossible for me to stand up to authority. I knew in those moments that I, we, had lost any argument for non-intervention. In any case I had felt all along that I was more in favour than Rick of letting nature take its course.

In spite of the appearance of choice, we really seemed to have very little at all.

It hurt to hear it said that if I hoped the baby would die I might well be wrong. But it was true. I hadn't wanted to give my own baby a chance in this life because I couldn't cope with its deformities. Had I such a right? Had I the right to choose for someone else? I don't know. All I knew was that these things, while they might not be so bad for a baby, would become increasingly difficult and complex as the baby became a child, as the child became an adolescent and the adolescent an adult, with an adult-size body. Then, I knew, this human being, at present no more than a few pounds of life, would be a full-grown individual with the most awful problems any person could be asked to cope with: no real sex, no sex organs, no normal life, possibly unable to go to the toilet normally, unable to have an adult relationship, unable to marry. It seemed a heavy load to be starting life with and this individual, I felt too, might well turn around and accuse us of having given it this awful life

For now, though, I knew my selfish thoughts were uppermost. The devastating effect on my own life, on our life, on our relationship, on our other child, was uppermost in my mind and it seemed too much for me to cope with. If God was not to blame then Francis was. We were the cause of Francis. Our act of love had conceived this abnormality, this aberration of nature. God had allowed it to happen and Francis, simply by being, was the cause of all our misery. It was a circle of responsibility and blame that never ended but went on and on, round and round, endlessly, hopelessly inconclusive, generating more and more guilt in me.

That morning, though, more immediate issues were at stake.

I left that consultation feeling terribly upset and angry. When the surgeon had left Sr Anna spoke briefly to us. I can't remember anything she said but I know I resented her even more and I was very much aware that she wanted us to agree to allow them to do all in their power to help Francis. The surgeon, I felt, had read my position very accurately. No matter what way I turned or twisted this baby was simply not going to disappear. Strangely enough, it was not the argument that they might lose time by delaying surgery which most swayed me but the mental steps from agreeing to feed, to agreeing to treat the jaundice, to agreeing to antibiotics if they were needed. There was no clear firm line where you could stop. I could never, ever have agreed that feeding should be withheld from the baby but neither could I withhold treatment for something that might cause brain damage. Once I took that second step I was already starting to acquiesce to aggressive treatment of a condition; antibiotics, too, would have been almost impossible to refuse.

I kept hearing my mother's words: 'Wouldn't the little thing be better off dead.' She, of all people, had, I felt, the right to say that. For her sake, partly, I felt I should put up a fight for my views. Now I felt both defeated and angry that we had only an illusion of free choice.

The other major change was that Rick had been completely won over and felt we should immediately agree to allow them go ahead with preparations for surgery. I refused to make any decisions there and then. (My father did always say I was stubborn.) I said I wanted time to think and talks things over and would not make any decision without sleeping on it. I suppose this was sheer stubbornness when, in my heart of hearts, I knew I'd be saying the same as Rick the following morning. However, I felt at that moment that I needed to go home, just with Rick, away from that hospital.

So we went up to see Francis. The violet lights were on, the blindfold was on: the treatment was continuing. The nurse asked if we would like to hold Francis for a few minutes. I still didn't want to particularly but agreed. Everything I did or did not do, everything I felt or did not feel, it seemed, was a source of further guilt to me. I was in terrible turmoil and ashamed of myself but I could no more change the way I felt than I could change the colour of my hair.

Deftly the blindfold was removed. Reverentially Francis was wrapped in a green, hospital blanket, and we took turns holding this tiny morsel of humanity which was the source of such soul-searching and anguish in our lives.

4

IT'S A GIRL!

We had talked some more about the situation at home. I had conceded that we should go ahead and let them operate. I still felt that I was cornered and not making a free choice. I still cherished the fantasy of bringing the little baby home, minding it by the fire – even keeping it warm in a drawer or something, like you read about in novels. But this was the twentieth century. Instead of a fire and herbal remedies there would be monitors and drips, sterile dressings and ultra-violet.

We drove over to Crumlin, once more ready to present a united front. We got the impression that the consultant was relieved about this. At one meeting he actually said that at least we felt the same about things. Some parents obviously didn't. Sr Anna could not hide her delight about our decision. Her enthusiasm and her kindness to us were almost infectious. I was certainly far from ready to share her enthusiasm but there was a small element of relief in giving up my crusade to allow nature take its course. I had felt I would be fighting the whole establishment, and, ultimately, going against what Rick wanted.

The consultant said they could now go ahead and plan for the first operation and that it might even take place that Friday or over the weekend. He again stressed that it was a long road ahead and that our baby still had about a fifty-fifty chance. He said the condition was so rare that it was difficult to be exact. Between them, the relevant surgeons in this country had probably dealt with about five such cases. One of them, he said, was now doing very well. We never heard exactly what had become of the others.

Our next consultation with him is the one that I will always remember with the greatest mixture of emotions. Once again Sr Anna was present. It was one of the few times in those early days that I felt something akin to happiness.

He told us the test had shown our baby to be a girl. I could hardly believe my ears! Now we had a label; now at last the baby was really a human being because it had a sex. Now we had a pronoun. And a girl, what I had wished so hard for! It seemed to solve so many problems, most importantly the fact that we would now be able to bring her up with the sex she actually was. We would not, after all, be required to live a lifelong secret lie.

I heard him say they had thought the baby was probably a boy as these problems tend to occur more often in boys but that they could be wrong. The test was not the only test they could do and was not infallible. He said they could do another test but it would more than likely have the same result. I heard all that and took it in but discounted any small doubts. After all, they themselves were telling us the second test would almost certainly have the same result. In my delight, I hardly noticed Rick's feelings. He had really believed our baby was a boy.

To me, this was the first good piece of news we had heard. Frances. Now I could call her by her name. Frances.

When we got home we phoned my parents, Rick's mother and Denise. I was enthusiastic on the phone. I felt almost alive again. Rick was less happy about it all. After all, he was having to make a major adjustment although he did agree with me that it solved the problem of bringing the child up as a girl if it was a boy.

'Sex not determined', the pink label put on Frances's wrist and ankle at birth, was no longer true. We had a girl. For the first time since the birth I felt I would be able to talk to people about our baby. Yes, she's a girl, a little girl. Frances.

Rick's mother arrived in Dublin and we both collected her at the airport. Our neighbour once again looked after Stephen, who was now almost back to his normal self. We went straight to Crumlin with Rick's mother and, for the first time, she met Frances, her seventh grandchild. I know she was really moved with love and tenderness when she saw and held her. She also felt so deeply for us and for our sorrow. It was a long, long time later before I began to appreciate, to any great degree, just how much our parents grieved for us and how very difficult the situation was for them, doubly troubled by their grandchild's problems and by our grief and stress.

Sr Anna told us that the operation had now been provisionally arranged for Monday. Frances was not exactly thriving, however. She had lost weight and was now barely three pounds. Her face seemed more pinched and old-looking than ever. She was still being treated for jaundice although the nurses always tried to take her out for us to hold for a short while when we visited.

One young student nurse, in particular, already seemed to have taken a liking to her.

When we called to my parents later, my father, almost shyly, expressed a wish to see Frances. I was really pleased. I hadn't wanted to suggest it as I knew he could be very squeamish about things. As the operation was now scheduled for Monday, we agreed it would be a good idea to try and arrange for both my parents to go in to see Frances before that, my mother's condition permitting.

On Saturday morning I announced that I was going to go to

the hairdresser and get my hair cut. I thought it would be a positive thing to do and might make me feel better. Rick's mother asked me if I'd like her to go with me but I said no, that I'd be fine. So off I went. I felt slightly strange as I had hardly driven at all in the previous few weeks. It was a bit like the feeling you have after flu when you're still a bit weak and washed out and the world seems at a remove from you all the time.

I parked in the car-park of the shopping centre. I suppose I was barely five seconds from the car when I began to feel totally out of my depth. This was the first time I had been out on my own since the baby's birth. On top of that, this was the first time I'd been anywhere apart from a house or hospital since the birth. It seemed such a long time, nearly like another life, since I had come to this place and done normal things like shopping. But much worse than that were all the people. There were people everywhere, hurrying, holding their children's hands, wheeling buggies. It was a typical Saturday morning but all I could see everywhere were children, more children, lots and lots of normal, healthy children. It was almost unbearable. I hurried along and up the stairs to the hairdressers and sat in the queue for hair washing. Somehow I got through that. But when they put me sitting down in front of a mirror to wait for cutting I broke down. I started sobbing quietly there in the middle of the salon. They didn't know what was wrong with me. They asked me if I was all right and gave me paper hankies. I couldn't start explaining to them that I'd just had a deformed baby and it was in Crumlin and I didn't know what to do. So I just sat there and cried and got my hair cut and fled.

Rick went in to see Frances with his mother and I stayed at home. There was really no change in her. Everything in us was now focused on this operation, a huge hurdle for such a tiny human being. Fifty-fifty were the odds; that stuck out in our minds.

So, there I was at home, a seemingly normal mother with a normal, healthy baby. And that dark cloud over me. We were both so glad to have Stephen; to come home to him. He was our 'Exhibit A' so to speak, our proof that we could have a normal baby. He was the baby that was ours to handle, to feed, to cuddle, to play with, whose nappy we could change. We were also very glad that he was too young to understand most of what was going on, but already I had thought ahead to the awful possibility of Frances's living for a couple of years, coming home and of Stephen's becoming terribly attached to her and then losing her. That, I felt, would have been harder even than any sadness I might have had myself. I hoped Stephen would be spared that.

That weekend I believe I made significant progress in 'bonding' with Frances. I was so delighted with her being a girl that I felt I could cope better with the physical abnormalities. Also, I suppose, there was a certain relief in having decided to take one road as opposed to another; her future lay in the surgeon's hands.

The nurses had suggested to us a couple of times that we might like to take some photographs but we decided not to. We still had the awful photograph from the night of the birth but we both thought we would wait until after the operation before taking that step.

Because Frances had been so premature I had bought only two things before the birth. One was a blanket exactly the same as the one I'd bought for Stephen and which became his security blanket. The other was a little gown. When Stephen was born I noticed that one of the mothers in the Coombe had used gowns instead of Babygros and I thought they looked so sweet I decided I'd get one for this baby. Now that Frances was a girl it seemed even more appropriate to use it, so I decided to bring it in with me that afternoon and ask the nurse to put it on her.

My mother and father came with us to the hospital. We had phoned in advance to check if we could use a wheelchair from casualty to bring my mother up to the ward. The nurses were, as always, helpful, and knew it was an important visit for us, not only because Frances's grandparents were being introduced to her, but also because the operation was to take place the following day. Both my parents held Frances that afternoon and the nurse put the little gown on her and admired her in it. Even my mother, who was frail and small herself, had no bother holding the little figure, so light, in her arms.

While we were there, a junior doctor came and told us that Frances's electrolyte levels had dropped significantly and that she would need to go on a drip to bring them back up, particularly as the operation was scheduled for the following day. He told us it would not be able to go ahead unless this had been righted.

I suppose that was the first setback but it wasn't conveyed to us as an emergency or anything; it just left us with a slight doubt about the operation.

My father took my mother home before we left because her tremor came on. Rick and I waited for a little while and then said our goodbyes to Frances, very aware that she would be out of our hands, literally and metaphorically, for the next twenty-four hours.

It was that afternoon when it first dawned on me, watching Rick's tenderness and love for this, our second child, that no matter what happened now: whether she lived or died our lives would never be the same. She was here now and Rick loved her and if she were to die on the operating table the following day Rick would always feel her loss And if she lived – then there would be so many more complications, operations and decisions. The thought left me feeling defeated.

We phoned the hospital, as instructed, at nine on the following

Monday morning, only to be told that the operation had been postponed: Frances's electrolytes were not quite back up to the right levels and she needed to stay on the drip a little longer. It was a letdown. We felt deflated. So much emotional energy in the previous four days had gone into preparing ourselves for this momentous surgery. I even felt the goodbyes the previous afternoon had been wasted – they were for something that now wasn't going to happen yet. We could go in to see Frances again that afternoon.

Rick decided that, as the operation had been postponed, he might as well go into work the following day. I know it was a real effort for him and that his mind was far from work. I have never, before or since, seen him so reluctant to go to the office. I know that he, too, found it difficult facing people. Even facing sympathy *en masse*, seeing people who wish you the best in the world, can be terribly difficult when you feel so low. However, he did go in on the Tuesday and that broke the ice for him.

On Tuesday the nurses said the operation might go ahead the next day. We kept the possibility of another postponement in mind and talked about 'if' not 'when'. Once again the nurses told us to phone the hospital the next morning to find out if there had been a definite decision. Once again we said goodbye to our little girl and went home to Stephen.

5

FIRST OPERATION

On Wednesday, 3 February Rick phoned the hospital and he was told the operation was going to go ahead later in the morning. He was to phone back in an hour or so and they would tell us whether Frances had gone into theatre.

We got the breakfast; we tidied up; we did everything mechanically that morning; and we were so keyed up that we talked very little.

Rick rang the hospital again about ten and we learned that Frances had left the ward for theatre. He spoke to Sr Anna and she suggested he phone back in a couple of hours when she might have some idea of how the operation was going. She also told him that she would ring us about half an hour before it was due to finish to give us time to be there so that we could speak to the surgeon afterwards.

Our tension increased immediately, knowing that Frances was going to theatre, knowing what the odds were. Anything could happen. It was going to be a long day.

Not long afterwards a friend of mine, whom I hadn't seen since before Frances was born, called to see me, presuming I was still pregnant and simply wanting to know how I was keeping. She was obviously stunned by what we told her and embarrassed to have called while we were in such a situation. I can remember her sitting on the sofa and feeling for her. But I was just not able to say or do anything to change the atmosphere. She did not stay long and we were once more left to our own devices, rattling round in the house with only Rick's mother, like a rock of common sense, to keep us calm.

Still, I played intensely with Stephen that morning. He had a favourite toy at that time – he'd got it for Christmas. It was a set of interlocking cups which could be stacked into a tower and had six or eight shapes for posting through the lid. Every morning he made for that toy and took all the cups out, rolled them, dropped little cups into big cups, poured shapes from one cup to another and then distributed everything all over again.

Another car pulled up. This time it was the district nurse. She was a really good nurse: practical and conscientious about checking out the babies and mothers in her charge. She was obliged to call on me, having been notified through the system of the birth of Frances. But once again, as if from a far-off distance, I pitied her that day, having to call on us. We were a difficult case, I could see. It's a bit like having some sort of social leprosy.

Frances's operation was a colostomy, which would mean she would have a bag on the outside of her body to take the matter from her bowel and so keep it separate from the urine. The idea of a colostomy did not seem all that bad to me. I certainly did not feel it was the hardest problem to deal with. After all, she would have known nothing else. A bag for urine, I felt, would be much more problematic and the prospect of nappies for six or seven years was also fairly daunting. The nurse had agreed that that could well be the case.

But at least she was a girl and we could bring her up as a girl. I still had that to comfort me. If she died on the operating table or shortly afterwards, so be it. We would have to cope with that if it happened. Still, on balance, for me the nightmare would be over if that were the ending this evening or tomorrow. But I also had the tiniest seed of optimism inside me that I could, perhaps, learn to love this little girl and cope with her problems. It might be too soon to talk of love yet but there was at least a spark of feeling there now where for a week there had seemed to be no sign of anything.

I went on playing with Stephen. Mrs Boyle sat in the chair and listened to the radio. Rick read his book – it was about the first successful ascent of Everest. Sir Edmund Hillary battling against the elements. There was no adult conversation and even my interchanges with Stephen were fairly quiet. But we were all intensely alert and jumpy. The time passed painfully slowly.

Eventually Rick felt he could phone again. We were told Frances was still in theatre and likely to be there for a couple of hours longer. Again we were told Sr Anna would phone us as soon as there was any indication that it was nearly over and then we could come in straight away. But for the moment, we were advised, we might as well stay at home.

We made lunch. I have no idea what we ate. I normally enjoy my food but all through that time I simply ate because it was mealtime and I knew I had to eat. Also, that day, it helped pass another half hour. We have a red clock on the wall in the kitchen. It's fairly quiet but when there's no noise you can hear every second ticking with a slight, plastic sound. That day we each felt all those thousands of seconds individually.

I got Stephen up again, fed him and changed his nappy. The poor child. I nearly cried every time I thought what all this might mean to him, how, although he didn't know it, his life too, had been utterly changed in the past two weeks. No, not his life, but his future. There was nothing at all I could do to change that for him. And I desperately wanted to.

I played with Stephen for a while. Arrangements for Sir

Edmund Hillary and Tensing were proceeding nicely. Rick and I hadn't discussed what either one of us would do that day or how we'd pass the time but as both of us seemed best able to do what we were at we left each other at it.

Finally, finally the phone rang again and we all jumped. Rick answered it. Yes. OK. We'll leave straight away. Sr Anna had told him the operation should be over in about half an hour. It was about half past three. We said goodbye to Mrs Boyle and put on our coats, conscious of our hearts beating away. We said goodbye to Stephen and went out to our car.

The drive to Crumlin that day seemed to take for ever. Give or take a yard or two it was ten miles from our house to the hospital. But it was a dark, grey day and the traffic was heavy. We trundled through Milltown, Terenure, Crumlin village. It was about twenty to five by the time we were finally climbing the stairs to Holy Angels ward. Sr Anna had told us to call in there and see her first.

The first let-down was that we were too late to see the surgeon. He had waited, Sr Anna said, as long as he could, but then had had to go to attend to another commitment. But we could see his registrar. Yes, we said. I felt angry at that straight away because we could have come much sooner. What a waste of time – our sitting at home.

Frances was in Special Care, she told us, and had come through the operation as well as could be expected. The registrar would tell us more about how things had gone. She showed us into a small room. We sat down and when the registrar came in Sr Anna left. He introduced himself to us with great emphasis as if we were most unlikely to remember his name at this, our first meeting. He pointed the name out to us on his badge. It stuck in my mind for ever.

He began by explaining to us exactly what the procedure had

been and the aim of it. But somewhere along the line, very soon, in fact, while realising that this man was articulate and good at explaining, I could hear something else; I could feel something huge coming. I stopped hearing the sense of what he was saying altogether. All I could feel was this huge thing coming at me – he kept talking about 'your baby'; not Frances; no 'she's; just 'your baby' all the time.

Now in the case of your baby, he said. And then the storm broke. Another test and tissue they had found during the operation, both showed the baby was a boy. He said he knew that the previous test had shown the baby was a girl. But . . .

Long before he got to the end of the first sentence with the first indication in it of this shocking change of sex I was howling loudly. Sobbing, crying. I was completely out of control. I don't know what else he said. I heard only one thing out of that entire discourse: I had lost my baby girl. Now they were telling me it was a boy after all. It was too much. The earlier test had, after all, been fallible.

At some stage the registrar said goodbye and left us and at some later stage Rick left the room and I heard Sr Anna saying, 'Is she very upset?' Then she came in and put her arm around me and said how sorry she was and how she, too, was upset about it.

Upset was too mild a word to describe me. I was inconsolable. I still cry when I think of that afternoon. I really felt my world had ended and I hated that baby. I really hated that baby of mine.

Then I was standing in a corridor. I can't remember whether it was upstairs or downstairs. I was thinking that if I had the courage of my convictions I would go into Special Care and take the baby and run away. I thought that if I drove to Dun Laoghaire I could get the 8.45 sailing from Dun Laoghaire to Holyhead, that I could use my Access card to buy my ticket. I thought the baby might well die on the journey but that if it did that would be for the best. And if I was charged so be it, but the police would probably put it all down to postnatal depression or something and even if they didn't I didn't really care. I thought that whole plot out like that, standing in the corridor. I kept telling myself to go in and grab the baby and make a run for it while I stood there rooted to the spot and did nothing.

Then another thought occurred to me: You made the decision to go ahead with the operation. You gave your consent. So now you can't just withdraw it and give the baby no chance; you've got to stick to the road you've taken. You have allowed the surgeon to use his skills to give your baby a better chance in life. You can't just violate that chance now.

I don't know how many times in the next couple of days I still wished I had stolen the baby and made a dash for the boat. It had seemed a terribly plausible and sensible thing to do at the time. Now it just seems bizarre but it does show how crazily mixed up I was and how close I was to cracking up altogether.

Rick went in to see Francis. I didn't want to and would not. We left the hospital. I cried all the way home in the car.

When we got to our estate I said I would go in and tell Margaret. Rick asked me several times if I was sure, if I was up to it, if I wanted him to go in with me. I assured him I would rather go myself.

I got out of the car and rang the doorbell. Margaret opened the door, took one look at me, threw her arms around me and started crying herself. I vaguely wondered how she could possibly have heard the news but mistakenly judged by her reaction that she had, so I thought no more about it. She brought me in and sat me down and I blubbered and made occasional comments and we both cried again. Margaret says I was there for fifteen or twenty minutes and then I left and she said if there was anything at all we wanted just to call them.

I went into our house and cried again and sat miserably in the sitting room and more miserably in our bedroom and let Rick deal with everything: the phone calls to his sisters and my sister and the several other friends who rang enquiring. And no matter where I was in the house I could still hear Rick telling them all that now our baby was a boy, not a girl, and more tears would come and I couldn't stop them.

Mrs Boyle said it was no harm to have a good cry but this cry of mine seemed to have no end. At some stage in the evening a chance word made something click in me and I said to Rick that maybe Margaret had thought the baby was dead. He jumped up and said he'd go straight down to her just in case she had thought that but I couldn't see why it was so urgent. I really wasn't reacting normally to any situation; my judgement was way off.

He ran off down the road and came back to say yes, that Margaret had thought the baby was dead. I realised we'd been at complete cross purposes all the time I'd been there because I'd obviously been so incoherent I'd managed to say nothing at all.

We went to bed and got some sleep. I stayed in bed the next morning and cried again. Rick got Stephen up and phoned the hospital. They told him Francis had got a bit tired during the night and that he had been transferred to Intensive Care, where he was on a ventilator just to help him with breathing. So our baby was fighting hard. The surgeon had been so skilful that he had brought that tiny creature through hours of delicate work, had been successful and had given this little life a fighting chance. Yet I didn't care where the baby was. I wanted so badly for that baby to die.

Rick brought me up my breakfast and left me alone for a while and I just sat there, in bed, with no intention of ever getting up again. It's really unlike me not to want to be with people or to talk about things but that morning I just wanted to turn my face to the wall and die myself. I did not want this boy and now we were back to the awful dilemma: would they make us bring it up as a girl?

Eventually Rick came up to me again. 'Don't you crack up on me now,' he said. I said I wouldn't. He said maybe I should get up and I said maybe. I made an effort and told him he could start worrying about me when I stopped crying because that would mean things were really bad with me. He said he'd remember that. He told me about Stephen and then he brought Stephen up to me. Between them, they started to bring me back from wherever I was heading and after a while I did get up. I got dressed and went downstairs. I said hello to Mrs Boyle. I had cried so much that I didn't cry then for a while but inside I was still sobbing to break my heart and it didn't seem to be doing me a whit of good.

In the afternoon we drove back over to the hospital. A bright, cheerful nurse came out of Intensive Care to us. She introduced herself to us by her first name and said she was looking after Francis today. I hated her. I hated her cheerfulness. I hated Intensive Care. You have to wash your hands and put on plastic aprons before you go through the second set of double doors and then when you go in you look only for your child. You see nothing else. You don't want to see the rest. You've more than enough on your plate already.

Francis had quite a few tubes and drips attached and someone had put a tiny little white hat on the nearly-bald head which looked really odd considering there were no clothes at all on the little battered body which still had the energy to breathe and stay alive despite everything.

The nurse told us Francis was sick. We subsequently realised that that, in Crumlin, was a euphemism for 'seriously ill'. But, she said, he was breathing himself.

That should be *her*self, I thought. Yesterday it was *her*self.

She said he was the best of all of the babies in there and, she thought, would be the first out, meaning back up to an ordinary ward. But they had taken away my little girl. This baby, this body, was once again a complete stranger to me. I was back at minus ten and still hoping this baby would go back to where it had come from.

We didn't stay all that long. In Intensive Care they don't encourage you to. The nurse said we could come back in again later for a few minutes if we wanted to but that he was doing fine and that we were to feel free to phone them at any stage if we were worried, even if it was the middle of the night; there would always be someone there and they didn't mind. She asked us if we would like to see a doctor before we left and we said we would.

A house doctor was sent up to see us. He also worked under the surgeon. He was not as descriptive or talkative as the registrar and he did not, as the saying goes, 'have a great way with him.'

He gave us to understand that things were not nearly as clear-cut as we had been led to believe the previous day. He was much less certain that Frances/is was a boy: 'That's the plan at the moment,' were his exact words, 'But it's not a black-and-white situation.' He said the best they could hope for was to keep the child dry with a catheter. So we really were back to the boy-but-bring-it-up-as-a-girl-scene.

We left. We had not touched the baby. Even touching requires permission in Intensive Care. We took off the plastic aprons and put them in the black sack provided, pushed open the heavy double doors and went back out on to the landing.

During the drive Rick suggested we stop somewhere for a coffee. It was a good idea. It seemed really strange sitting in the coffee shop. I felt we were out of place among all these normal people doing normal things. I felt that we stuck out a mile although of course nobody would know just by looking at us that we had a baby with no sex lying up in Intensive Care in Crumlin on a ventilator.

We did actually manage to have a short talk over that coffee. Rick commented that I wasn't crying. I smiled ruefully and said, no, but that I wasn't as bad as I had been the day before. I asked him how he felt and he said he just felt numb. I asked him how he felt about Frances/is being a boy now. He said he didn't mind all that much because he had thought he was a boy all along and so it had been stranger for him when they had told us she was a girl. He'd found it harder to adjust to that. Poor Rick. I felt I hadn't paid enough attention to his feelings after that shift in circumstances because I'd been too intent on celebrating the fact myself.

We agreed that we had to see the surgeon because if, at worst, he put another position to us entirely, at least his was most likely to be the authoritative one and we would have three then to compare with one other.

So we went home again. Rick rang the hospital and got the surgeon's secretary and she made an appointment for us to see him the following afternoon.

Then there were more calls to our house. We saw Stephen and Mrs Boyle and we went to bed again and we woke up again the next morning and nothing had changed. Rick rang and Francis was still in Intensive Care but doing very well and would possibly be taken off the ventilator later in the day or the next day.

Rick went off to work that Friday morning. Another week was almost over. He came home at lunchtime. Stephen was still fairly cranky but better all the same and I was able to give him a lot of attention because I wasn't able to concentrate on doing anything useful around the house.

Rick drove us the ten miles to the hospital again. We arrived there half an hour earlier than the appointed time so we sat in Intensive Care beside our baby's place. It was not a bed. It was more like a large table up at an angle with drips attached and the electronic monitor blipping away. That's the noise you hear when you go into Intensive Care, the noise of machinery, not of people or conversation.

The nurse chatted to us once again and we touched the baby's hands. The little cap was still in place and the body still looked very tiny and white and frail, and I still did not feel any surge of love for this, a part of myself. The nurse told us that it's believed babies that small don't feel pain in the same way as adults. Anyway, she assured us our baby was not in pain.

Eventually she went away to check whether the surgeon was going to see us. She came back with the news that he had been called away to another hospital to see to an urgent case. She said we could see his registrar if we liked.

The registrar came up again. It was a very different interview from that on the Wednesday, the day of the operation. He was very cautious that afternoon. There were no certainties now about the baby being a boy; he was not definite, as he had been previously. He said we would really have to talk to the surgeon about it all.

Rick told him that if Frances/is was a boy then we would like to bring him up as a boy.

He told us he would pass that on. I know he wanted to reassure us. I know he would have if he'd had the authority to because he was a very warm, communicative person and from these very first meetings with him I quickly got the impression that he was genuinely interested in our child.

We left Intensive Care. We went out on to the landing and down the stairs, past the painted house and along the corridor, past the little shop to the porter's desk and front doors, out into the air and down the steps into the small, overcrowded car-park. Now we were faced with a whole weekend in limbo.

I did linguistic somersaults that weekend that twisted my mind.

I avoided the words 'he' and 'she' like the plague. I referred to 'the baby' and sometimes to Frances/is but I also managed to make sentences that skated past gender altogether. It became a challenge, almost an outlet for my bitterness. Once or twice I used the word 'it' but felt that was really wrong. It's all right to call an unborn baby 'it' and parents often do; but once birth has visibly defined the baby as he or she, what normal mother or father would ever again refer to their child as 'it'? But we were left in that dilemma. I felt I could have no relationship with an 'it' and until I knew what we had up there in Intensive Care there was no chance of any relationship forming. On the contrary: more and more I felt I had given birth to a monster and I felt deeply ashamed of the baby on top of the guilt that I felt no love.

Frances/is was still in Intensive Care when Rick phoned the following morning but had had a good night and was expected to be moved later in the morning. The nurse he spoke to suggested that we ring again before coming in to visit to see if the move had taken place.

I phoned at lunchtime. It was the first time I had phoned the hospital since the operation. Perhaps the shock was wearing off and I was coming back to life myself. The nurse I spoke to in Intensive Care seemed at first not to know who I was enquiring about but then she said: 'Ah, was that the little chap in the cap?' I said it more than likely was and she went off to find out more.

Our baby, she told me, had been moved to Special Care about an hour previously. She asked me if I knew where that was. I told her I did. Special Care had been my introduction to Crumlin Hospital and, I suppose because it was the first place I'd been, I was glad we were going back there.

Rick's mother and I went in to the hospital that afternoon and Rick stayed at home with Stephen. It was an awful visit for me. I don't know what I'd been expecting but of course the simple fact of moving from Intensive Care to Special Care did not mean there had been a miraculous recovery. Although weaning off the ventilator had been successful and relatively quick, this was still a very small baby who had been through major surgery. Before the operation Frances/is's weight had been dropping. We'd been assured that losing some weight immediately after birth was normal but we all knew that it had gone beyond the normal weight loss. There had been no gain: this was a baby of fractionally over three pounds in weight.

It must have been decided by the doctors that feeding should be started. It was now Saturday and the operation had been on Wednesday so this was the fourth day without any feeding. I had never known before, but subsequently learnt, that very young babies can actually lose the instinct to suck and feed if they are fed intravenously for too long.

It was about half past two when Rick's mother and I arrived. A young nurse I had not met before was looking after Frances/is and one other baby. She seemed a bit flustered when we came in. It transpired that she had given Frances/is this first feed and it had all promptly been vomited back up. She had just finishing clearing up the mess and settling things back to normal. We took our positions up beside the incubator, which was over beside the window, and spoke in to Frances/is who with fewer attachments at least looked more like a baby. There was still a drip-site left in as a precaution in case a drip was needed suddenly and there was still the wound but we had been told that that should heal up well. You could see the colostomy now, with the plastic bag for faecal matter. Separating it from the urine was intended to reduce the risk of infection.

The nurse sat on a chair with a table in front of her and began writing up her notes. After a few moments she asked me if I knew what sex the baby was yet. I told her it still wasn't definite. She said the notes had been referring to 'she' but had changed to 'he' in the past few days so she said she might as well continue on with 'he'.

That short conversation really upset me although I did not cry. I felt really angry and defiant inside. After all the differing views we had heard and our unsuccessful attempts to see the surgeon, I was not prepared to say Frances/is was a boy or a girl until I had been told which in very definite terms. Until then I would live in limbo. While there was still the possibility of being told we had a boy but had to bring it up as a girl I would not say anything definite to anybody.

I was also angry that here we were, two weeks and two days after our baby's birth still with 'sex undetermined' as the wrist and ankle labels had put it at birth. It seemed unfair that so much time had gone by and we still had no answer. We still had an 'it'. I was also feeling resentment towards Frances/is for doing so well, for still being in my life. That's a terrible thing to say and I felt guilty too, but I cannot honestly say that I felt anything good towards our baby that day; I hadn't since the operation. It was as if another baby had replaced ours because this was no longer the girl I had begun to feel affection for. It may seem childish to have such a need for a label, for a pronoun, but whenever I went over that in my mind I came back to feeling that it wasn't unreasonable. I couldn't deal with an 'it' because a person's sex is probably the first thing you establish when you meet or speak to anyone. It was knowledge I needed before I could begin any kind of relationship.

When we left I felt pretty disheartened. I told Rick what had happened and again he said we'd just have to wait until we saw the surgeon.

The next day, Sunday, Margaret looked after Stephen while the three of us went again to the hospital but when we got to Special Care Frances/is was no longer there. Special Care had been very busy, necessitating a transfer to Holy Angels. We trooped into Holy Angels. The staff nurse there was lovely and showed us into the little glass cubicle where our baby was. Everything seemed stable. Frances/is had come a long way in three days – from ventilator right back to an ordinary ward.

Finally on the Monday morning we got to see the surgeon and finally we seemed to have a definite sex for our baby. I still kept thinking of the surgeon's argument that we were dealing with intelligence and wondering whether it would not be better for our child if he were also slightly mentally disabled. The disabilities would somehow seem less acute because they would not have the same repercussions and we would not be striving to give the child as normal a life as possible against terrible odds.

Anyway, that morning my mind was focussing on sexual identity. The surgeon told us he had just been speaking to his colleague again and that he had confirmed with him that the child was a boy and that was that. We asked if we would be able to bring him up as a boy. He told us yes. So, in two short sentences, our world was substantially altered yet again. I had definitely lost the girl for good but at least we would not now have to live a lie.

The surgeon said he was sorry for all the trauma and that perhaps they had taken us through some aspects a bit too fast. He told us to put that behind us now. It was all over in less than a minute. I didn't feel any of the gladness I had felt when I was told we had a girl. But it was nice to re-establish some kind of certainty again after the previous five days of limbo.

The rest of the information from the surgeon was much as we had expected. The operation had been a technical success, he told us, and Francis had done well, apart from that first night after the operation when he had given cause for concern.

I asked whether there was a likelihood that he might have to wear nappies for years. Yes, he told me, that was possible, but he suggested that we shouldn't look too far ahead at this stage. He said it was going to be a long road.

He told us the large bowel was very short, which would make any reversal of the colostomy difficult and that a second operation would still be needed to try to close the bladder. He also told us that Francis' chromosomes were male and that they had found evidence of a penis and testes during the operation.

There was a certain relief after the consultation. At least I could stop calling the baby 'it' now. 'He' was now the official word. The thought of what would have been written on the birth certificate if we had been told to bring up the boy as a girl had tortured me. My mind could still hardly cope with the thought of that prospect and now, at least, that awful vista had been removed. So long as they didn't change their minds again, so long as they were right this time . . . For a long time afterwards I still had doubts. I would look at our baby and wonder. I would look and at times I could still picture him as a girl. Then I would look at other babies and realise that if you were told what sex they were you would accept it. I realised that many babies are indistinguishable when they are small. It's only because you have been told or that they are wearing pink or blue clothes, that you 'know' that babies are male or female without actually seeing them with their nappies off; and it is only because of that information that you 'see' them in a certain way.

Well now at last we too had a baby with a label the world could understand.

6
LETTERS I

January 25
Dear Richard and Mary
I can't tell you how sorry I was/am to hear of the difficulty with your baby.
My thoughts are with you both and I hope you will find the strength and
hope to sustain one another over the next few critical weeks.

For my own part, all I can say is that it is possible for a family to
live with a handicapped child and be happy and fulfilled — it just takes
that special effort and caring which we are all capable of when the
chips are down. None of us can predict the future unfortunately — just
hope that whatever happens, it will be for the best.
Take care of each other and Stephen.
Love
Evelyn

January 25
Dear Mary
I've been thinking of you constantly in these last few days, at this very
difficult time for you. I know well how worrying the 'early days' can
be. Take plenty of photos of your little baby . . . I know I appreciate
now having clear memories of the difficult days.

I hope I can visit you soon.
Love
Nollaig

January 27
Dear Richard and Mary
Just a few lines to let you know that you are in our thoughts and prayers. It is difficult to find any words of comfort but can only send our heartfelt love to all of you. Frances is only one week old, and is already a much loved member of our family. I just wish I could be there and have those lovely long fingers grip mine and stroke the little blonde head   Those precious moments will be with you no matter what the future brings. Stephen must be a great comfort to you during this time, also quite a handful by now, I should think. You must take good care of yourselves. You need to keep rested and healthy for both your babies. Put your trust in God. Live life one day at a time. We love you all very much. Give our love to your Mum and Dad, Mary, and a big big kiss for Stephen and Frances.
Love and prayers
God bless
Barbara

Dear Richard and Mary
Just a few lines to let you know that we are thinking of you all during this difficult time. We are all praying that the doctors can do something for the baby and in just a few short weeks all will be joyful for you. Please give Stephen all our love.
Sincerely yours
Joe

February 5

Mary

Talking to you last night, Mary, I don't blame you going back to calling the baby 'it'. It is a really difficult situation. Thinking about it, I reckon some of the doctors probably want to wait until the bladder operation before deciding whether the baby is a boy or girl. I hope you don't have to wait that long but if it was for the baby's welfare, then I suppose you'd have to. However, it would make taking the baby home even more difficult. That was an awful misunderstanding with Margaret, also.

If I were you, I wouldn't want to face knowing I was going to have a baby which required such an awful lot of care in such a delicate area as well as knowing I hadn't produced the normal healthy baby. Yes, I'd feel envious of that woman in the ward whose baby died – better to have nothing than a baby that isn't all right. And people say so much can be done for children nowadays in the way of operations. When I was with you that weekend and people were positive about the baby, it was quite distressing. You don't want to believe the awful change in your life the baby will bring you – or you feel at present, it will bring you – but I think if you start to care for the baby you would begin to see it more as a person – even if you didn't feel too maternal. Don't worry about this, just now – I think the sex situation is really difficult – but you'll get help and I think you'll probably find other people to talk to, with very similar feelings to what you have at present. I think it is so awful that you have to go through this, both of you, but try and take the baby a day at a time. Gradually you will accept it more if it does live, almost despite yourself.

May write another letter before I post this. Will see.

Love, lots of love

Denise

February 11
Dear Richard and Mary

I'm sending these for you to have because when I found this prayer some time ago I thought that it was a nice one for a new baby. Of course it's for all of you too, but especially Francis, and when you have it with you it'll remind you that someone is saying a little prayer for him.

Mary, who called the day when you were here, sent me a lovely card and when I spoke to her tonight she said to tell you that they were thinking and praying for you. All my friends have been really thoughtful. Give Stephen and Francis a kiss from me. Mum says Stephen's getting about quite well and nearly working up to venturing on his own.

Love to you all
Marie-Therese

February 19
Dear Mary

We are so very, very sorry to hear about poor little Francis. It must be a truly heartbreaking time for you both. As you say, it must be impossible to understand why it should have happened to you. Life seems so cruel and confusing at a time like this. Please God he's not in pain.

Thank goodness you have Stephen. The fact that you have one lovely, healthy baby must be helping you a bit.

Of all my friends, Mary, I have always felt that you were by far the strongest, mentally, and the most balanced. I pray that that mental and moral strength won't fail you now and that you will find the courage and strength to battle on in these very sad circumstances. I only wish there was something I could do to help. Even if I lived in Dublin I could be available for babysitting, but being so far away I can't even offer that.

I do so hope the news will get better about Francis. We'll keep praying hard.

We're both thinking of you all. Lots of love and a kiss for Stephen.
Love from
Paula

February 26
Dear Mary and Rick
I now feel that I can write to you and send you both our congratulations on the birth of your second son. I have hesitated writing to you before because of the problems but understand from Denise that you are both now much happier with the situation.

We are all very sorry that Francis has these problems and sincerely hope that medical science will be able to perform a miracle in the very near future. Don't give up hope or let the problems get you down. I'm sure you have many friends you can turn to for support and guidance.

We are all thinking of you and look forward to seeing the four of you very soon. I hear your news from Denise so feel we haven't lost contact.

Time to go now. All the best to everyone.
Love
Chris and Sue

February 22
My dear Mary
Thank you for your lovely letter. On the day it came, I was feeling rather sad, My house felt very quiet too, with Marie Therese back at work, and I was missing you and Richard and of course Stephen. You were in my thoughts all the time, (and still are) and so very specially is my youngest grandson Francis. I do wish I was near enough to be able to see him, however, as next best thing plant a kiss on him from me, and you had better give Stephen one too. We don't want him to feel left out.

From what I hear Francis is still putting up a brave fight, and I'm sure if God spares him, he will grow up a very brave and strong boy. And if love will help him, he has loads of it coming to him from the whole of the family

I know that you are both strong enough and your love for one another is deep enough to cope with anything, hard though it sometimes seems. I hope Stephen has got rid of his cold, but he won't come to any harm if he is still sleeping and eating as he was.

I must finish now, and get some work done. The weather is quite good, so I have no excuse: I must do some washing!

My prayers and love from

Mrs Boyle /Marie /Mum

Take your pick!!

February 29

Dear Mary

A brief note hoping you are well. I hope and pray that your little son is getting better and that he'll be home with you soon.

You've probably heard that we had a daughter on February 4. She's very well; it's hard to believe she's four weeks old.

You are constantly in my thoughts and if I can be any help to you, please call me if only for a chat.

Mind yourself.

Love

Marian

7

ROUTINE OF SORTS

Over the next few days the confirmation of Francis being a boy and the permission to bring him up as a boy sank in. It was at least a relief to be able to speak normally about the baby – to refer to 'he' and 'his'. After a few tentative attempts I began to gain a little more confidence.

I had at one moment while talking to the surgeon felt he was just the slightest bit impatient with my preoccupation with our child's sex. It barely showed. It seemed that, for him, there were more pressing and urgent problems; he simply emphasised that our baby still had severe problems and that trying to sort out his bowel and bladder would be their priorities. I never believed he understood how I felt.

To me, without a sex the baby was a nothing, and it hardly mattered what else was wrong. Other flaws would receive no consideration until this matter of sexual identity was established. If the baby died, I would face the fact. If the baby lived then it was more urgent to get that vital element sorted out. In my view no physical problem could compare with having no sex. I could imagine someone asking what was wrong with the baby and wondered how I might respond. But before that point always, always, always I knew that the first question would be: 'Is it a boy or a girl?' or 'What did you have?' If I couldn't get beyond that . . .

I knew that people all over the world have to cope with various deformities of various severity but I had never heard of anyone who had not started out as a boy or a girl.

But just as Francis's becoming a 'he' sorted out this huge difficulty it also confirmed others: he would never be normal; he might never be able to excrete normally; he would more than likely be sterile. There was still a long list of problems. I worried at them and turned them over in my mind, day after day. I used to wonder if there would ever again be a day when I didn't cry.

In spite of the trauma and continuing worries things slowly started to return to some kind of normality in that we began to establish a routine in our lives.

Two days after we saw the surgeon Rick's mother went back to England. Rick was also back at work full-time now. The day after Rick's mother left I took Stephen down to the babyminder's and drove to the hospital. It was only when I got there that it struck me that this was my first visit alone.

I just sat in the glass cubicle in Holy Angels ward and looked at my little baby and cried. I couldn't stop. The nurses were always very sensitive to things like that and a young trainee nurse soon came in to me. She was already fond of Francis, you could see. She told me I shouldn't feel ashamed of him, that he was stronger than almost any other baby on the ward. She was enthusiastic. She told me you could see his strength by the way he moved around and kicked. She said you could tell fairly quickly when a baby was a fighter and she was sure Francis was. And, indeed, at just over a week since his operation you could see the improvement and healing already.

The nurse wrapped him in a hospital blanket and took him out of the incubator and let me hold him. It was the first time I'd held him since the operation. Holding and being held are central to the parent/child relationship. Putting your finger through a baby's fist is no substitute. Holding Francis was really important.

However, the sister on the ward also told me that day that Francis was not feeding well. It wasn't just a remark such as mothers would make about their baby; it meant more. On the other hand it wasn't long since the operation, which must have affected his digestion to some extent. There was still a good chance that things would improve so that Francis could start putting on weight.

The following day Rick went to see Francis and I stayed at home with Stephen. It still felt both strange and fraudulent being at home on maternity leave with no baby but on the other hand I did need the time and I still felt physically drained myself. It was also nice for Stephen to have me there for a few months

When he got back to the office after his visit Rick rang me to say that Francis had vomited again. So no improvement on the feeding front. Still we had staggered through another week and we were a good deal less traumatised than we had been seven days previously.

Margaret had asked us if she could see Francis; so on the Sunday we all went in: Margaret, Don, Rick and I – and Stephen. We decided it was time that he too met his little brother, now we knew it was a brother he had, and we had checked with the nurses that that would be all right.

Margaret and I went in together. Francis was lying in the incubator not looking too bad, I thought. He did have a tube from his nose which led down into his stomach so that any feeds he didn't finish himself could be syringed into his stomach by the nurses. I realised that in spite of everything I had got used to seeing him. Margaret on the other hand was upset and we came back out fairly quickly. She said it was that he was so small and even though she thought she knew what to expect, the sight still came as a shock. It might seem strange but Margaret's tears made me see that I had made some progress towards adjusting to the situation. I certainly didn't feel I was doing fine or anything – far from it. I was still a morass of mixed feelings, resentments, sadness, anger and pity but . . . I *was* getting through each day.

It wasn't after all one of the unhappiest of afternoons. We let Stephen peep in at Francis. He really didn't seem to take it in that there was a baby there at all. He was far more interested in the incubator than its contents but at least this was something other parents did – show their new baby to their firstborn. We felt confident enough, too, that weekend to take some photographs. The nurse wrapped Francis up in a blanket and we took turns holding him. Don even took a photograph of the four of us together.

Looking at those photographs now I can see how pitifully thin and small Francis was – as small as a doll, really, and about the same weight, with a pointed wizened little face. Yet at the time he didn't look so bad to us.

The following day Francis was moved back in to Special Care. I was told he needed to gain some weight and so it had been decided to put him on something called Total Parenteral Nutrition – complete intravenous feeding. TPN as it was called for short would give Francis all the proteins, carbohydrates, minerals and so on that he needed straight into his bloodstream without his having to use his digestive system at all. A few days of that, it was felt, might build him up sufficiently and then they would try the feeds again.

I was not unduly upset by the move. We were back in Special Care, after all, where Francis got such good attention. It was a temporary thing which he needed and could well give him the boost necessary to establish the feeds again. In the meantime, soothers or dummies were the order of the day. The first thing a baby gets when he/she is admitted to Crumlin, I think, is a soother and it became Francis's greatest treat in life. At that stage, however, he was still not able to keep it in his mouth and it was always falling out.

We had been thinking and talking about Francis's name. I was not happy with it. Now, if he was to be a boy, I felt he needed a male-only name. While Francis had been a wonderful way-out in the early days, being ambiguous, I felt it was unfair to leave him with it for fear it could become a source of teasing in later life. With his problems I felt he needed a unambiguously male name.

We thought of several and at one stage had even decided to call him Conor but then put the subject back into the melting-pot. Then Rick suggested James. He said it was a good family name because his late father had been called John James and my father's name was James Anthony. We both really like it. My father was vehement that he didn't want the baby called after him – he could sometimes be funny about the most surprising things – but we assured him that he wasn't the only source, so he agreed.

We then had to tell Sr Anna. I knew it meant extra work for her. She admitted it but she also understood our reasoning. Now everyone had to get used to the new name, including ourselves, and it took a few weeks for people to adjust. We left Francis as his second name because it was part of him too and so he became James Francis. My father's rueful comment was that his name was now bigger than himself. I was really pleased with it. Ever since I'd lost Frances and she'd become Francis I had felt ill-at-ease with the name: it had belonged to the girl but didn't sit well with the boy. So James it was.

Our friends were good to us. We had been sent a lot of letters as well as cards and Mass bouquets. A couple of friends waited until it seemed certain that James was a boy and then gave us 'boy' presents and 'boy' cards. I really appreciated the thoughtfulness of that. Other people seemed unsure whether to offer sympathy or not.

The public health nurse called again. I had to tell her that Francis was now a boy called James and she, I suppose, had to change her records again. She repeated that survival was the important thing for the time being. I also had to ring the VHI again to change his name to James, after Francis and Frances. Well, third time lucky. If it was the same person I was speaking to each time, she must have thought we were fairly stupid and indecisive parents.

Lent began that week but I just didn't have the heart to do anything. Giving up sweets or chocolate seemed to me a trite thing to do at the time. I was also still at odds with God. I blamed him for devastating my life. I railed at him in my mind: what did he think he was at and why did he hate me so much as to do this to me/us. Wasn't it enough that we'd had to watch my mother suffering for years with Parkinson's disease without this as well? Whenever I went to Mass I ended up crying. Everything I'd believed in seemed terribly childish now. Adversity certainly hadn't strengthened faith in my case although I did say prayers at times, particularly the Memorare, a prayer I have always liked, on the basis that Our Lady could hardly be blamed for this almighty mess. And look at what she'd had to put up with!

James was on TPN for four days and he did gain some weight. The doctors seemed pleased with him and so on the Friday of that week he was moved back into Holy Angels, which was just across the landing from Special Care. Sr Anna said she could see the difference in him. She said he'd been fading away in front of our eyes before the new treatment.

The following Tuesday James was moved back into Special

Care yet again – his fourth admission there. He hadn't sustained the weight he'd gained on TPN the previous week; he still wasn't feeding well and needed the TPN again. Sr Anna told Rick that this time he would be going on TPN for weeks rather than days. From the way she said it, and he relayed it to me, we both got the impression that this was fairly serious. As long as he was on TPN he would also have to be nursed in Special Care because this particular drip required constant monitoring and detailed checking, which meant it also required a lot of nursing hours.

Sometimes I would go in and find the nurse using a calculator to work out the figures for James's chart: what was going in and how much, as well as what was coming out the other end. She would check to make sure the drip was flowing properly, examine the bag of fluid hanging from it and then, when the highly-sensitive alarm on the drip went off, as it frequently did, come back to find the cause of the alarm and do it all over again.

James was also put on another little monitor, the size of a small transistor, which kept a check on his breaths per minute. That was another headache for the nurses as it was inclined to set off its alarm regularly, causing them to rush back to him, check him and reset it. After a while we got used to these alarms and realised they rarely, if ever, meant a crisis in James's case. In fact we would stand there rather embarrassed in case it was something we'd done which had set the damn things off in the first place. But that's just another example of how powerless we were. We could not do anything to tend our own child in those circumstances; we always had to rely on someone else to come and help us out.

When I went in on the Wednesday afternoon I met again a wonderful nurse, Nora, whom I'd first seen nursing James during his previous stint in Special Care. Nora was another person who helped me along the way towards feeling something genuine, something akin to love, for my own baby.

She could not let me hold him. He was too thin now to be taken out of the incubator or moved about much. Absolutely everything was being done to conserve his energy. He was lying on a tiny sheepskin rug, with just a nappy on, a morsel of humanity. Nora showed me how to put my hand in through one of the 'portholes' – the little round doors on the side of the incubator and stroke his head or hold his fist. Other people had also allowed us to do this but it was the way she showed me and her whole manner of nursing him which woke something in me. Here again was a nurse who did more than simply take care of the babies in her charge; she actually seemed to transmit a part of herself to the babies, to give herself to them.

I asked her how she felt James was. I knew, as I was asking it, that it was unfair of me, as nurses aren't really allowed to give detailed prognoses or predictions about their patients. The worst I ever heard a nurse say to parents of a baby was that he was 'sick'. I felt like rushing over to them that day, strangers as they were, and telling them that it meant their baby was seriously ill, perhaps verging on the critical, certainly on the point of being moved to Intensive Care. But of course I didn't, because you don't interfere; you don't intrude on other parents and their problems. You sometimes feel like the three wise monkeys hearing no evil, seeing no evil, thinking no evil, except that it is all pretence. There's very little privacy in a hospital but with other parents respecting your space and the invisible lines that mark out the patch around your baby, you survive. If necessary you ignore other people's tears and what you hear them being told, and they in their turn ignore yours. It's not being impersonal. Far from it. But all parents in Special Care are coping with their own acute problems and very often want to be left alone. You don't want other people prying into your business, and while you might strike up a conversation or even an acquaintance with other parents the discussion of the children stays at the most superficial level. It can be about soothers or toys or the weather or the drips or the baby's crying, if it's lucky enough to be able to cry and isn't on oxygen, but it's seldom about exactly what's wrong. The nurses, for their part, discourage enquiries about other babies.

However, that afternoon I asked Nora how she felt James was because I wanted to hear what she would say. We had got into the habit of ringing the hospital every morning to see how he was and how he'd been during the night but the news, the pronouncements were always pretty much the same. He'd had a fine night, he was fine or, even, he was in great form and would we be in later to see him? That would be the extent of it. That afternoon, I remember, Nora paused for a moment, as if she wanted to choose her words carefully and then she said: 'Well, Mrs Boyle, to tell you the truth, he just looks thinner to me than the last time he was here.'

It was a simple, obvious statement and yet it hit me in the face. Of course, he was thinner. I knew that already really because we'd been told he'd lost weight. But how thin could a baby get and stay off the critical list? It was clear from the way James was now being handled – what with the sheepskin, our not being allowed to take him out of the incubator and the TPN – that he was not at all well. It came home to me that afternoon, just as I started to feel something for him, how critical things still were.

Perhaps he'll die, I thought, even fairly soon. And then I'll be free again, free of all this terrible burden of worrying. He really could die. This all might go away like a bad dream. But even at that stage I knew it was never going to be that simple. I knew Rick would be heartbroken. I knew too that you just can't go back to where you were as if nothing has happened; you have to go on.

And anyway he probably would do well on the TPN, as he had the last time, so there would be no need to think of death or dying.

So the week went on. We were not in a crisis, exactly. No one was telling us things were terrible with James but we seemed to be holding our breaths all the time and the anxiety levels were back up. You could tell by how jumpy we were whenever the phone rang.

Then my father decided that he wanted to come in to see James again. That was fair enough. I agreed and arranged that he'd come in with me on the Friday. I was pretty sure the nurses wouldn't mind as they had allowed my parents in before, admittedly when James was on Holy Angels.

However, as soon as I walked in the door and saw James across the room I knew I had made a big mistake. I realised then that I should have left my father outside, gone in first myself and waited for a suitable time before bringing him in. I never brought anyone in completely unannounced again. James, unfortunately, had rolled over in the incubator and was lying at one end, almost up against the side of it. We could see him through it. As I said before, I was aware that he'd got thinner but I was used to seeing him every day. I had not considered the effect on someone seeing for the first time. In that moment, of course, I saw James as my father saw him and I realised just how very small and scrawny he must look. The impression was made worse by the awkward angle at which he was lying.

My father looked at him and I wasn't surprised to hear his reaction. 'Oh my God, Mary,' he said. 'There's no hope. He couldn't possibly stay alive. Just look at him.' And he went on in a similar, shocked vein, for several minutes. The nurse took in the situation immediately and quickly moved James, doing her best to make him look 'presentable' for his grandfather. There was not a lot she could do; she couldn't wrap him up in a blanket or take him out or hide his emaciation in any way.

I know that day shocked my father and he didn't ask to come in to see James again for quite a long time. When eventually he did he was just as surprised at the change in him as he had been shocked before and called it a 'transformation', admitting that he'd given up all hope of ever seeing him alive again after his previous visit.

The following Sunday afternoon, when Rick and I were visiting James there was a young couple in the room with us. I couldn't help hearing the nurse talking to them about their baby who, it became clear, had had some kind of stop-gap heart operation and was likely to be discharged from Crumlin within days.

The mother discussed her breastmilk and the bottlefuls she had expressed and what was in the fridge to feed the baby until she got in the next day. She and her husband cooed over their little one and showed their obvious delight and optimism about the whole situation. You could feel they were just waiting for a return to normality after this major hiccup and were fully confident it was just around the corner.

I sat very quietly looking in at our thin baby. Again I felt an almost uncontrollable anger, and envy of that young couple. I would have loved to shout at them: 'You think you've got problems? Come and look at this! Oh yes, you can sit there and talk about expressing milk and the rest. How would you like to have to cope with this?' I have never in my life wished so hard that I just had a baby with a heart defect: how simple: you operate, and it works or it doesn't.

Even going home in the car that afternoon I said it to Rick, how wonderful it would be if James had a heart defect instead of the problems he had. I don't think he quite saw it my way. He was much better at acceptance than I was; I hadn't even started.

It was now the end of February in a leap year. Stephen was going to be one year old on the Tuesday, the first of March. I was determined to celebrate his birthday.

It seemed incredible that he was only going to be one. We'd been through so much since James had been born that he seemed to have been on our minds for an awful lot longer than a month and a half. It seemed strange to be celebrating our elder child's first birthday with another child born and having been through major surgery. There certainly were many times during our first few years of married life when I just wanted our lives to slow down a little. Everything seemed to happen with such speed and devastation that it was like a boxing-match, with the two of us continually getting up only to be knocked flat on our backs straight away.

I spent the next two days trying to prepare a little family birthday party for Stephen. It sticks out in my mind for several reasons. A first child's first birthday is an occasion people never forget but of course this one had an added poignancy because Stephen had a baby brother in hospital ten miles away who was absent from the party. And, inevitably, it led to thoughts of whether James would ever have a first birthday party himself and, if so, whether he would be able to be at home for it.

On top of all these thoughts, still constantly swimming round in my mind, there was the sheer physical effort involved in rising even to this minimal level of entertaining in our own house. It seemed to take a monumental effort even to make a sponge cake and ice it, to get ready to greet my own parents with a few other guests, and get through a party. It surprised me, even at the time, how difficult I found it. But, typically for me, I pressed on. I was absolutely determined that Stephen should have his first birthday and that we would have photographs of it.

In the rather twisted way my mind tended to work at that stage I thought I was not going to let James spoil Stephen's first birthday. That, too, I would have laid at James's door if it had not come off. It was a bad lookout, I would say, for later stages, if James were at home and his poor health caused some outing or plans to be cancelled. Would I have gone on blaming him for it all? I don't know. I just don't know. Quite possibly I would.

Anyway, I visited James the day before the birthday and Rick visited him on the day. We have several photographs of a family group standing around Stephen's high chair as he blows out his single candle. None of them betray how we really felt at all. It all looks tremendously normal – perfect family album material.

Now it was March. James once again responded well to the TPN – no crumbs of birthday cake for him – and put on weight. He seemed to be out of danger in the matter of nutrition but went on to get repeated urinary infections which required antibiotics.

8

OUR LIVES

Things were undoubtedly better than they had been in the beginning. We knew we had a baby we could call a boy or 'he' and we had given him a name which we both liked. There were other things, though, which I also wanted for him. They were things that even I felt a bit shallow for seeking but they are important. Clothes and bottles may seem just outer trappings but where a baby is concerned they have a greater significance. Changing and feeding a new baby take up an awful lot of a mother's time and these things are intimately wrapped up in the whole process of caring for and getting to know this new human being. All the holding and cuddling and talking and getting-to-know that goes with doing those things are a vital part of the loving of the baby.

For the early part of his life James wore no clothes. In a heated incubator he had no need for them. He would be occasionally wrapped in a blanket and lifted out for a few minutes at most. So I could not dress him or even see him dressed up. I could not feed him either. The breastfeeding option was long gone and although sometimes he was fed by bottle, for days on end he might not be, because of diarrhoea, urinary infection or some other problem. Even when he was being fed the nurses gave him most of his bottles and the amounts were minuscule: they began with just 10 ml, the equivalent of two teaspoonfuls.

Then there was his hair. He had had a few blonde wisps when he was born but soon after he went on drips his head was shaved. The nurses needed more sites for locating the drip and the head was a good source of veins. As a result, James was permanently bald, his head shaved every so often, and that made me sad too.

We were almost totally powerless as parents: We could not lift James or hold him without permission. When he was very sick we couldn't hold him at all. Even when we were permitted to have him for a little while we had to be very careful as the the drip site might be in his head or his tiny leg be in a splint to hold the needle.

If we wanted to feed James we first had to make sure that he was on bottles, then time the visit to coincide with a feeding time or ring up to tell the nurses when we would be in. It was really frustrating to have done all that and then find that another nurse hadn't got the message and had fed him already. It was no one's fault. The nurses were extremely busy and they genuinely encouraged us to do what we could for James. They were disappointed themselves if one of us came in just as he was finishing a bottle.

Changing his nappy was a major task and the nurses did that too. Since the operation there was no big growth out from the bottom of his stomach but there was open tissue – it was a bit like looking at someone's insides with the skin sliced away. Then there was the bag. The area around it had to be kept as clean as possible to avoid infection. We could never walk in, lift James and change his nappy. We were also reminded, tactfully, to wash our hands when we arrived before even touching him.

On the plus side, James had beautiful eyes and, when he wasn't jaundiced, the fairest skin, almost translucent, like fine bone china. He also had delicate, perfect limbs. As time went by the pointedness of his ears became less noticeable and as no one had said anything to me about his hands or feet I presumed they must be normal and enjoyed them. Those fingers and toes were so perfect they were a continuous consolation to me.

There were people to comfort me too. My sister, Denise, kept in close touch. One of my sisters-in-law, Anne, who lived in Germany, was a physiotherapist and had worked in a children's hospital in England for several years. Not only was she knowledgeable but she was also very good at talking to me and turning over the situation with me. When she phoned I would stay talking to her for a long while and feel much better afterwards. Then there was Margaret, who became a firm friend. She had infinite patience with me whenever I knocked on her door and sat in her kitchen going over and over it all for the 'n'th time. She would still listen and still sympathise, pour coffee into me, then distract me and cheer me up.

James's feeding problems continued but he was no longer at death's door because he had gained weight on TPN. Bottle feeds were also necessary, however, because of the danger that he would lose his instinct to suck. We never got as far as solids with James but it was a big day for each of us when we first fed him – holding him as you would any baby, in our arms, putting the teat into his mouth and watching some of it go down. It had to be separate days, of course, because we still only went in together once a week, on a Sunday.

The feeds, which started with what looked like just a dribble in the bottom of the bottle, would be painstakingly increased to 15 ml and 20 ml over the days. They consisted of an artificial substance, made up in the laboratory. We were still a long way from commercial formula feeds but it was progress. James might be on eight of these 10 ml feeds a day, being fed every three hours.

The feeds smelt horrible. In the beginning I really found that smell revolting but as time went by I got used to it and it became James's smell.

We learnt to read his chart which was a sheet of paper with about ten headings on it giving information on temperature, weight, amount of TPN being administered and his output in millilitres. The nurses would have to measure the amount in his colostomy bag and the figures would be compared. When the amount coming out at the far end exceeded the amount going in in oral feeds then things were not good. It was a very delicate balance. I got to the stage where every time I arrived in his room I would check his weight and his output and that gave me a fair idea of how he was.

One afternoon, out of the blue, I asked if there was a social worker in the hospital that I could see. The nurses seemed slightly surprised but readily agreed to ask her to see me. Although I had been a public patient in the Coombe we were in the VHI and so James had been admitted to Crumlin as a VHI patient. I had been worrying about the VHI cover for him and even though the nurses had indicated that they thought it would not be a problem I wanted to clear up the question once and for all.

The social worker, whom I met a couple of days later, told me James would be covered for six months under the VHI and would then become a public patient. But, she told me, he would get the same care and be in the same cot or on the same ward whether public or private. She also told me, which was very reassuring, that Special Care was completely funded by the state anyway because it came into the same category as Intensive Care and was a public facility. On a practical level that was all good news although, unfortunately, about seven months later the hospital sent me a bill for thirteen thousand pounds. By then, however, that was a minor problem in the general scheme of things and I just passed it on to the VHI and told them I didn't care what happened, that they could deal with the hospital.

The social worker also reassured me that we were not alone in having a child in the hospital long-term. She said there were other patients and parents in the same position as ourselves. She also suggested that we might like to meet James's medical doctor. We, of course, had been totally ignorant of the fact that two separate departments were closely involved in James's case. While the surgeon had been in full charge of the surgery, the TPN and medical care of James was in the hands of another doctor.

We duly met her in her room one afternoon, together. It turned out that she had been involved in James's treatment to some extent from very early on. However, she said, she had felt we'd had enough to deal with talking to everyone else and so she had not suggested a further consultation with her.

She went on to ask about our other child and about how we had been coping emotionally. She asked us if we had reacted by not wanting to hold the baby. I think I misunderstood her and thought she was talking about Stephen. So I assured her that, no, that was in no way the case. Looking back on it I think she may, in fact, have been talking about James and so I missed the single opportunity that presented itself to open the floodgates to a professional and confess that, yes, I hadn't wanted to hold him, touch him, have anything to do with him and was still struggling with all kinds of confused feelings and thoughts about him. But the opportunity was lost.

She ended her chat with us by telling us to enjoy him. I think it took me about two years to really understand or appreciate that remark. That day it just made me feel angry. I felt like retorting: 'How do you think I can enjoy this baby that doesn't function properly, can't feed, can't be dressed, can't be taken home and barely has a sex? I knew she meant well, so I said nothing. We smiled and thanked her and left.

At home, when I'd put Stephen up for his morning nap and hadn't an awful lot to do but far too much to think over, I often used to cry. The tears just kept coming – day in, day out. At some stage in February I felt so worn out crying and so fed up generally that I concluded it would have been better if I had never met Rick. I had questioned it before but that one day I really believed it – I felt I would give it all up just to be out of this nightmare I was in, that I'd really rather be lonely and on my own than go on with this. I only remember being that bad on one morning but the tears didn't stop.

I found some particular situations triggered them too, being on my own, at Mass and listening to nice music. Occasionally people's sympathy would be enough to make me disintegrate into a damp mess. As a consequence I got so embarrassed with crying at Mass that I stopped going every week and just went when I felt up to it. I was still feeling fairly angry with God at times. At other times I would be driving – usually to or from the hospital – and a nice song or even a piece of classical music would be enough to bring on tears and I'd have to turn off the radio.

Rick never cried through all those months, not once, but the strain told on him in physical terms, too, and he looked more and more worn out.

I used to quail inside whenever I thought of minding James at home. The responsibility would be awesome between his three-hourly feeds and his colostomy site – keeping it clean and changed and free of infection – never mind the worries about whether he was getting an infection or running a temperature as well as all the normal colds, infections and teething that everyone has to deal with in a perfectly healthy child. I knew we would be perpetually tired. Mind you, we seemed to be perpetually tired even with a team of nurses caring for our child.

Another aspect of the situation was that I would have to give up my job if James came home. I had asked our babyminder would she be prepared to mind him eventually but I did so as much out of courtesy and to review my options as out of any expectation that she would, or should, take on such responsibility. As I'd expected she said no. Once I rang a nursing agency but the rates charged for a nurse in your home were absolutely prohibitive so that was also out of the question.

I'm sure many people feel I ought to have wanted to give up work and have been glad to pay such a small price for having James home but in those early months of shock and confusion it seemed to me one more huge sacrifice that I would be asked to make. I had worked since I was twenty and enjoyed my job. I also knew that James would require a great deal more than a normal baby in terms of doctors visits, drugs and various other medical bills. I wasn't at all sure about how we'd cope financially or how I'd cope with being a full-time mother. I was loathe to make the decision. It was also another grudge, for want of another word, to lay at blameless James's door.

Rick and I, as a couple, outwardly coped extremely well with the strain. We talked over all the major decisions together and presented a united front to the doctors when we had to meet them but we are very different in personality and we were at different stages of reaction for that entire year. We used to say it was lucky that we were different. Whenever one of us seemed too tired to go on the other usually felt a bit better and could take over for a while – making dinner, putting Stephen to bed or visiting the hospital.

On an emotional level we were also different: Rick seemed to accept the situation far better than me. With absolute faith he said that whatever happened we would cope – together. He also loved James from the start and this quickly became a deep, unqualified love. As time went on I don't really think he believed James would die. He knew, because he'd been told, that there was a chance, but he didn't think about it all the time.

I was an emotional wreck from the moment this second baby of ours was born. When he was several months old I asked a qualified nurse who lived near us if she had any books that I could consult about some of his problems. She lent me some textbooks but warned me they were very technical so she wasn't sure how much good they'd be for me. I read all about bilirubin or jaundice, and the various treatments, and about other problems premature babies can develop. I glanced through other chapters and then I came to one about grief and it explained so much to me. It went through six stages from shock and disbelief through anger, bargaining with God and finally to acceptance. It also said a mother mourns the loss of the perfect baby she'd been expecting, particularly if, in any sense, she envisaged the baby as 'a gift' – for her husband, other children or parents.

The description seemed to fit me so well. I could identify with those early stages and definitely mourned the loss of the perfect baby I hadn't had, while trying to come to terms with the imperfect baby I had given birth to. It even went some way towards explaining the sense of shame I had about James and the feeling that I had somehow let Rick and Stephen down. It certainly made me feel slightly less abnormal than I had done.

But the circular thoughts still vexed me. Every day I lived out James's entire life in my head – from what it would be like when he came home to how he'd manage to start school, to the likelihood of readmissions to hospitals and operations for years to come. Worse than that was when I imagined other children's comments and their possible cruelty towards him, how he would cope with his adolescence and, worst of all, when he became a man and what he might feel then – a man unable to have a normal relationship with a woman perhaps, unlikely to be able to have

111

children in any case and a man with an awful, hidden disability, possibly needing two bags also for his bowel and bladder. It was always when I got to the adult stage that my mind would give way and I would despair. I could hardly bear to think about it and yet I couldn't stop thinking about it.

It was all very well dealing with this tiny baby; since all babies had nappies he wouldn't seem so very different. The thought of James as a fully grown man with all these problems was really too much for me. Sometimes I used to hope so hard that if he did come home and Stephen grew to love him and know him as his brother he would not die. I didn't know how I could bear to see Stephen's heart broken. At other times I used to pray that he might be allowed to enjoy a little of his childhood but that God would take him then, before the adult problems should appear. If he didn't live beyond childhood then maybe we would have made him happy enough for a few years. At other times again I still used to hope that he would die, for my sake, for his own sake, for Stephen's sake. I never hoped he would die for Rick's sake because I knew that in hoping for that outcome I was hoping for what would devastate Rick. There were no solutions and I felt I had absolutely no control over anything.

With regard to Rick and me as a couple, life was also changed. We seemed to live almost in separate shifts. When we were together we were nearly always tired. The only time we were together with James was on our joint weekly visit to the hospital.

I remember particularly one Sunday evening being allowed to hold James and even getting to feed him. After a while – which I hadn't felt was all that long – Rick asked me when I was going to let him hold James. It was nearly as if we were jealous of each other because on most visits we had him exclusively to ourselves.

So we had less time together than before and less energy to do anything outside home, work and the hospital. Our social lives had shrunk anyway because of two close pregnancies and having a young baby at home. Now social life virtually disappeared. We still loved each other but we were both very sad people. Occasions like Valentine's Day and Mother's Day seemed terribly inappropriate to our situation and merely accentuated our sadness. Just a year previously I'd been so proud of being a mother on my first Mother's Day. This time I was certainly not proud, and it was not a day for celebrating.

On the other hand I felt extremely lucky most of the time to have married such a good, consistent, loyal man with such strengths and such compassion. I really felt I could not have survived that time without him. Without a doubt he helped me to carry on and helped me to form a relationship with James.

Both our families did everything they possibly could to support us but it hurt that all of them, apart from my parents, lived in England while we were in Dublin.

On 22 March, I got a phone call to say that a good friend of mine had been found dead. Jim! I couldn't believe it. I'd last seen him when he'd called out shortly after James had been born. I went through the funeral because I had to but it was another shock that I felt ill-equipped to deal with. It seemed another senseless, inexplicable tragedy.

One afternoon when I was in visiting and chatting to the nurse who was tending James, another nurse joined in the conversation. Reacting to something that was said she looked me straight in the eye and told me, with firm emphasis, that James would not be going home for a long time. I was taken aback. You know that nurses are more aware of how things are with their little charges on a longer-term basis than they will concede when you ask how things are on a particular day. So this was an unusual statement, almost like a warning. I didn't want to read too much into it but it was said with great conviction. The nurse, whose judgement, I must add, I greatly admired, went on to say that another mother who'd had a baby in Special Care had been able to split her maternity leave and keep a good bit of it for when her baby did get home. She said if I was thinking of going back to work I should consider enquiring whether I should do the same.

This opened up new possibilities. There was no reason why I couldn't go back to work. I would still be able to visit James as often as before and have almost as much time at home with Stephen. Within a few days, after talking to Rick about it, I decided I would enquire as she had suggested. The response was quick and positive. I was told I could arrange to split my maternity leave and come back sooner than required so long as I had a certificate of fitness from my GP and my own department agreed to the arrangement. After that it was just a formality.

The very idea of returning to work gave me a boost. I began to feel I could return to the world, to *my* world, and possibly live my life something like I had before. Then if I had to give up work later, when James came home, it wouldn't seem as bad as if I'd never gone back. I seemed to need to cling desperately to my job.

There were definite neuroses too. I was over-anxious about Stephen. I knew it and yet I couldn't seem to stop it. I also had a terrible, gnawing fear that our house was going to go on fire. It used to come at me at bedtime in particular and build up into a major fear. Again I knew that was irrational but it wouldn't go away.

An analyst would, I'm sure, have a field day with it all. I suppose they were various manifestations of my sense of threat and insecurity. It was as if I were waiting for yet more disasters to happen, and the worst disasters I could envisage were something awful going wrong with Stephen's health or the house burning down. It extended to Rick too, one particular day. He had decided to have a game of golf and, taking the afternoon off, had gone to the local public course. I had no idea how long it would take to play a round of golf but vaguely thought about two hours. By the time Rick had been gone four and a half hours I was nearly sick with anxiety.

James went on making progress. I couldn't believe it one day when I went in and he was no longer in the incubator but in what they called a glass cot because it had perspex sides on it. Soon he was put in an ordinary hospital cot with metal rails. He looked absolutely tiny in it but he was out in the ward now and able to start taking in his surroundings.

People who enquired about him thought it was wonderful news that he was out of the incubator, as if that solved all his problems. They seemed to think the next step would be that he could come home and that he must now be thriving. It was difficult to explain that his problems were still as serious as ever, and, for the most part, I didn't even try. It just brought home to me again how little people understood, apart from those closest to us and how isolated we were – totally immersed now in the hospital but knowing no one else with any comparable problem.

Even the parents we did get to know, although they obviously had children with serious problems too, all had different problems to us and I remember one day when I did compare James with another baby, who'd had a colostomy reversed, a nurse was quick to emphasise that they were very different cases and I shouldn't compare them.

The nurses asked us if we had a baby bouncer and we brought it in. Sometimes when we went arrived James would be propped up there in his bouncer, dazzled and confused by the coloured balls in front of him which, every so often, his hand would touch.

He was also being dressed now, which made him look much more like a real baby, and he loved being held. The nurse used to say, 'Oh here comes Mum' and say this was what he wanted. I felt they were just saying it to me to make me feel good. I really didn't think James would know me from any of them at that stage; in fact it was several months more before I was sure he recognised me at all. But he certainly did enjoy a cuddle. The nurses used to say, 'That's what he'd like all day – just to be cuddled and walked around.' But really I knew he was still getting only a pathetically short amount of cuddling and conversation compared with a baby at home.

Then one day a nurse suggested to me that I might like to bring in some clothes for James. I did so on the very next visit and they were put in his locker and I was promised he would be dressed in them the very next time he was changed. Of course I never saw the clothes again. The nurses didn't distinguish them from any other hospital clothes. They were just thrown in with the rest of the laundry.

It was a bad start but I learnt. Another nurse suggested that I put his name on all his clothes and she would tell the others that he was going to be dressed in his own things. They could put the dirty ones in his locker for me to bring home. That started to work quite well.

I even began to feel like a proper visitor, bringing in clean clothes and taking the dirty ones home from the locker. At last I was doing something practical for my own baby, washing the little Babygros and hanging them out on our line at home and then seeing him dressed in the clothes I'd got ready. That gave me a real thrill. Several people, when they heard, bought clothes for him and he soon had a nice little wardrobe in addition to all Stephen's baby clothes. We got presents of a couple of outfits specially designed for premature babies and James looked really cute in them. They were so tiny and yet he hardly filled them but he looked magnificent all the same. I was really grateful to the nurse who'd suggested it because it was just what I needed.

At home, Stephen was taking his first steps. That was a real joy to watch. Tentative at first, he was soon clamouring at the front door to get out on the path and totter round the estate. It became a nightly event. He was full of chat and babble mixed and he was getting more teeth. Stephen really was our security. It was so wonderful to have another child at home, a healthy child with a good appetite and who was still young enough to need cuddles himself. How much worse to have only one, sick child, like many parents did or to have your first child born with terrible problems. At least we knew we could have a healthy child and we could leave Crumlin and go home to him.

One of the most popular songs that spring and summer was 'Don't Go' by Hothouse Flowers. It was being played everywhere. It became like a theme song for me.

First Rick, then I on the following day, were told that James had smiled. It took us another few days each to see our first smile but it was just breathtaking. James's smiles began in his grey eyes and gradually moved down his face until his mouth broke into the gayest, most laughing smile you could ever see while his eyes nearly danced in his head. This gave us another purpose to our visits: to get James to smile!

9

EASTER AND AFTER

Towards the end of March James was moved out of the three-bed room to one on his own. He had a virus and was in what they called 'isolation'. One of Rick's sisters, Barbara, was coming over that weekend so I hoped that she would still be allowed to visit.

They allowed my father to visit briefly with Rick and me one morning. My father was pleasantly surprised when he saw James this time as there was such an enormous improvement in him. His face had filled out, he was in a proper cot with gold hospital blankets over him and he was wearing real baby clothes.

Whenever James had an infection (or 'virus' as it was officially termed that time) we worried a little more. We would go back to ringing the hospital every morning to check how he'd been overnight and to hear what the house doctor had said on his round. The nurses always reassured us, giving the kind of information we wanted: he was sitting up in his bouncer, he had had a bottle, he was still in isolation.

We were in one of those anxious phases when Barbara and Joe arrived on the Sunday evening with their youngest son. Earlier that day Rick and I had visited the hospital together. The mother of a friend of mine lived very near the hospital and I had asked her if she would look after Stephen for us while we were at the hospital. Stephen had never 'made strange' before. He seemed uneasy when I handed him over and burst into a loud cry as I was leaving the room. We went on to the hospital but I just could not concentrate on James. I kept thinking of Stephen's cry and wanting to rush back to him.

I arranged to go back to work on 11 April, a week after Easter. That still left me with four weeks maternity leave and the option of an extra month without pay to take at some future date. It was now Holy Week. On the Wednesday a parcel arrived from Germany for Stephen. It was from Rick's sister there, Stephen's Auntie Anne. Inside was a beautiful soft toy for James, a bright red elephant which played a tune when you pulled a cord on it. There was a birthday present for Stephen, too, and a chocolate bunny for each of them.

Later we went down to visit my parents and managed to clear up the kitchen a bit. My mother was not well enough to do anything in the house any more and my father was not a good housekeeper. He admitted as much himself but hated my doing anything in the house. It was a regular bone of contention between us. His only concessions so far had been to allow a woman to come in once a fortnight to hoover and do some ironing, and he unwillingly took the Meals on Wheels I arranged. My mother ate hers but I knew he nearly always threw his in the bin. The situation at home was far from ideal.

Rick suggested that we should both have a weekend away. He said it would do us good to have a break but that, as one of us really had to be in Dublin we'd have to go separately. He said that I should go over to Denise and Ken for the weekend of the London Marathon in April. It was a great idea and I felt really tempted, especially as both of them were running that year.

I decided that we should paint the sitting-room. It badly needed it as it hadn't been done since the house was new. I knew if James came home any thoughts of decorating would be put off for a long time. Rick was less than enthusiastic about the idea but I went ahead and bought the paint.

On Holy Thursday Rick and I went up to Crumlin together. James had a urinary infection now, we were told. He had had a blood transfusion a few days previously because they felt his blood count was low and he was going to get another one that evening. It wasn't great news, any of it. After noticeable progress and what seemed like a brief time of near-equilibrium, he seemed to be slipping back again. James's progress had been real but not substantial. He couldn't afford to slip back.

Good Friday can be a bleak day at the best of times, which was another reason to keep busy and do something constructive. So, reluctantly but resignedly in the face of my determination, Rick helped me to empty the sitting-room while Stephen crawled around us, pulling himself up on the furniture every so often and quite enjoying the activity. Rick said he'd do the ceiling first while I took care of Stephen. After lunch he set off for the hospital.

I was sitting reading to Stephen when Ciaran arrived – he's the priest who married us and a good friend. He was studying in Rome and was home just for Easter. He produced a huge bouquet of flowers from the boot of the car and asked how we all were. I showed him into the chaotic kitchen and I told him all about James.

Soon after he left, Rick arrived back and got paint on his good jacket removing a spider at my insistence. This did not make him any more keen on the decorating job but we persevered. Things were back to normal by the following evening and I felt we were ready now if James came home. That afternoon I went in to see him. He was out of isolation and back in the other room with two other babies and I was able to feed him.

Easter Sunday was a good day for all of us. Stephen loved the chocolate bunny. We put on our best clothes and I even put on some make-up, probably for the first time since James had been born. The weather was beautiful, sunny and mild. My parents came for lunch and in the afternoon Rick and I had a lovely visit with James. We brought him in the presents from Anne, the musical elephant and the chocolate bunny, and a musical bell and matinee coat that Barbara had left for him. I had sewn a tape with his name written on it in indelible ink – that had become one of my occupations since he'd begun wearing his own clothes: writing out 'James Boyle' on the little labels and sewing them into his clothes. We told the nurses that they should eat the chocolate bunny but that as James had been sent it we wanted to bring it in to him. He seemed well and his eyes were really taken by the brightness of the elephant and the music. I fed him again too.

On the evening of Easter Monday Rick and I went to see James. My father was babysitting for us. I had felt really down that morning. I suppose the upbeat mood of the previous day had been too good to last and I was tired after the painting and cleaning. I felt when I woke up that I had the weight of the world on my shoulders. I was in a really black mood but after lunch we drove down to Djouce Woods and went for a walk through the sunny trees with Stephen. I felt much better after that. When we got home I sat on the back step, keeping an eye on him as he played around the wheelbarrow with stones and bits of dirt. There was still some warmth in the late afternoon sun and the world seemed less bleak again.

That night the hospital was very quiet and we had time on our own with James. He now weighed 2.88 kilos – nearly six pounds. Rick fed him that evening, rocked him to sleep and settled him into his cot. We knew he was content when we left though we often used to wonder how we would ever get him into a routine if he came home after the twenty-four-hour life in the hospital. We finished the weekend off by going for one drink on the way home.

On the Wednesday after Easter Denise arrived and that afternoon we had Stephen with us to visit James. We took turns holding my babies. Denise was really delighted with James and thought he was so different from when he was born. The nurses all admired Stephen and paid a lot attention to him. He'd only been in on two occasions before that so most of them hadn't met him before.

James wasn't so well the following day. Rick rang me after his visit to say he seemed to have his virus back and would be going into 'isolation' again soon. Apparently his temperature had gone up, although it was down again by the time Rick got in. By then he was peacefully asleep. I felt myself getting keyed up. For a few weeks things hadn't seemed too bad. When Rick got home, too, he said he thought James wasn't well at all. He also said he'd been taken off feeds again altogether.

I got a letter from work confirming my suspended maternity leave and the date for my return. In the afternoon I was asked to come back two days early and work the weekend. Reluctantly I agreed to work the Sunday.

James did not have a great night. When Rick rang first thing in the morning the nurse told him he was 'sick'. His temperature was up again and they had put him on another antibiotic. His white blood-cell count was up, indicating an infection, and so was his heart beat. He was in a tiny metal cot on a heart monitor. He was not being fed but neither was he on TPN. His only intake was glucose from a drip and antibiotics. His virus was back and he had a slight chest infection. The nurse remarked that he'd been through such a lot but he was a little fighter.

Denise had come with me in the afternoon. James was back in 'isolation' and the nurse was reluctant to let her stay in the room for the whole visit but she relented in the end. The next day James was much the same: his temperature was normal but he wasn't interested in his soother – a bad sign since that was usually his main interest in life.

On the Sunday James was half-asleep for most of the time we were there and still had no interest in his soother. He was asleep before we left – his heart monitor bleeping, his drips glunking and him oblivious to it all. Denise said that no matter what might happen James had had an identity and a personality. She and Rick left me out to RTE then to start my first day's work. It was harder than I had expected. The first person I met on the way in told me straight away that she was pregnant and she was obviously delighted with her news. The 'it's-not-fair' wail, the 'why-me?' went through me again. I wanted to turn round, going back down those stairs and ringing to say I had changed my mind: I couldn't face coming back yet.

I felt slow and stupid at my work too but luckily I didn't have a great deal of responsibility that afternoon and could just obey instructions. I went home at teatime so that I could say goodbye to Denise, who was going back that evening.

The next day I had to rush around to have all the chores done and get Stephen's stuff ready and bring him down to the babyminder – all by just after one o'clock! Since it was Monday there were far more people in at work. Lots of them came up to talk to me but luckily I felt stronger emotionally than on the previous day. I got off at seven. It was a lovely sunny evening. Poor little James – I still had such mixed feelings about him. He had vomited saliva twice in the morning but his temperature was normal and Rick said he was sleeping peacefully when he left.

The next day was bad. It stands out as one of the worst between James's two operations. I was working from two to ten o'clock but got off at seven so I was able to go to the hospital. The night shift came on duty while I was there and I met a nurse I had never seen before although she said she had minded James quite a number of times. She job-shared and opted for night work. She told me things we hadn't known before. Part of it was our own fault, I suppose, in that we had not pressed for more information but partly, too, there was a lack of communication in the system generally.

First she told me that James's jaundice was back and that the general infection he'd had in the past week was pneumonia. I was stunned. No one had mentioned the word pneumonia before. Chest infection was as far as we'd got. In my mental dictionary there was a big difference between the two. I began asking more questions then so she looked back through James's notes. She told me the official name of his condition – it consisted of two very unfamiliar words which I knew I would never remember. The point was it actually had a name – I had never realised that before. In addition, she told me, that when he was born he had a perforated anus and (another unfamiliar word) something wrong with his feet.

Now, with an array of complex problems like that you might think I'd focus most on the main condition or the jaundice – even the pneumonia. But I was really upset about his feet. Medically this was not regarded as significant. No one had told us he'd anything wrong with his feet. Those little feet, those toes that I had so admired, that I had comforted myself with for almost three months. 'At least his hands and feet are perfect,' I often used to think to myself. Now this nurse was telling me that wasn't so either.

She said splints and physiotherapy or arches in his shoes should correct it but I didn't care. I felt someone should have told us and that this was heartbreaking news on top of everything else. I know, of course, it was minor, a mere spot compared with James's major problems, but somehow they were so hugely overwhelming whereas this was something very tangible. It also meant I had to reconstruct my visions of James in the future: as well as possibly being doubly incontinent, he would also walk slightly oddly, or have to wear special shoes or arch supports. It was another huge sadness to me.

I stayed composed for the length of the visit but I cried all the way home and was still crying when I got there. I hadn't been as upset since the night of 3 February when I was told Frances was a boy.

While Rick was in visiting James the next day he happened to see the medical doctor and he confronted her, telling her we weren't getting enough information. I think he was angry on my behalf too, having seen me so upset again the night before. The doctor examined one of James's feet and said she could see nothing wrong with it but that she would ask the orthopaedic surgeon to have a look at him.

When I got home that night Rick again said that I should really consider going to London for the weekend, especially as I had Friday and Monday morning off anyway. Next morning I booked a flight to London for the following afternoon. That night when I went to see James I asked about his feet. The nurse said there might have been something wrong with them when he was born because of his foetal position but that they might already have corrected themselves. I thought myself that they looked all right.

I didn't mind travelling to London on my own. It was a reprieve, however temporary. I wouldn't say everything just disappeared for the weekend and I felt wonderful – my tortured mind was still with me – but I did benefit from being away. It was only the second time I'd been away from Stephen overnight since he'd been born, the first being when James was born. I rang Rick and heard that James was much the same, still not on bottles, but with a good colour and less agitated.

My return flight on the Monday morning was delayed for more than two hours, which meant that I couldn't get up to the hospital to see James before work. I got the car from Rick, though, and went up to see him on my tea-break. That, in turn, meant I couldn't get home at teatime to see Stephen. So when I got home from work that night I had to content myself with looking at him sleeping in his cot; he still looked like an angel when he was asleep.

That Wednesday when I went in the news was good: James was out of isolation; all the tests showed him clear of infection, his colostomy output was back to normal and even his weight was up, three kilos or six-and-a-half pounds. He was going to be three months old the following day. He was still a pound and a half lighter than Stephen when he was born but, on the other hand, with a lot of help he had actually doubled his weight since February. On the Thursday I got in to see him just as he was getting his first bottle in two weeks and I gave him the last drain of it. He immediately looked content and within a quarter of an hour started to drop off to sleep. God help him, on 20ml of half-strength chickfeed, as it was called, every three hours.

That Sunday we brought Stephen in with us to see James. He was still in very bad form but had no other obvious symptoms – no cough or cold or temperature. James, on the other hand, was in great form. When we got there the nurse said he had been smiling away at her just before we arrived. I was able to feed him and then Rick came up with Stephen. When the nurse saw we were all there she took James off the drip, put him in the ward's buggy and told us we could take him for a walk around the hospital.

It was a big outing for James – all those colours and new things to see. He seemed to be taking it all in, bright-eyed, and it was fun walking the two buggies along the corridors side-by-side. Luckily Rick had also brought his camera that day and took some photos. James was wrapped in an orange hospital blanket so no draughts would get to him, especially with his little head so bald, and he had the inevitable soother in his mouth. The walk made that visit a special occasion and for half an hour or so we were almost like a real, normal family.

Stephen was still miserable the next day. By that evening he had spots behind his ears and the next morning the doctor confirmed German measles. At least it was a relief to know that was all that was wrong with him

As Stephen got better I hit another bad patch. I suppose I was tired after the extra worry about his rubella. There were still plenty of days when I seemed to spend my time fighting back tears and when I could barely answer people's enquiries about James and how he was. Then James got another infection. I was crying in the car park of the hospital even before I got in to see him and when I did get in it was to be told that he was running a temperature of 101. It meant more antibiotics. He had lost interest in his bottles and was jaundiced again. Stephen, meanwhile, now had a cold and was teething.

We staggered on, our situation fully conforming to my father's axiom that life is a constant struggle.

10

SUMMERTIME

The evenings were starting to lengthen and it was bright now whenever we visited the hospital. The drive there never seemed to get any shorter. but when I got to the last major junction I could see the main building in front of me, pick out the window of James's room and know that in three or four minutes I would be up there with him.

One evening I was so fed up and confused that I blurted out at Rick that maybe they still weren't right, that maybe James was a girl. He was shocked. I suppose I didn't really think that any longer but I needed some way to show Rick how distraught I still was at times. We had a useful chat then about it all. He said he felt it was hard on me having to switch back to having a boy because I couldn't imagine how a boy would cope whereas he could imagine how he himself would cope if he had James's problems. But that wasn't the whole story for me. Firstly, I still thought it would have been much easier to make a girl look physically like a girl and to hide the abnormality completely – but only if the baby had really been a girl. Once it was a boy it was a case either of living a lie and bringing him up as a girl or else facing the prospect that the child would never be or even look like a proper boy.

The other thing was that with that switch from girl to boy I had lost the little daughter, Frances, that I had had for a week. The baby was still there and it was the same baby but 'she' was gone forever. I had even dared to think at moments that 'she' looked a bit like me. I never again let myself think that.

The first Friday in May when I got in to James he was very distressed – crying hard and lifting his head up with great energy to turn it from side to side. He had his nappy changed and I thought the wound was looking slightly smaller as his body lengthened. It looked longer that day and was bronzed too with the jaundice. When I saw how strong he was I thought: 'He will live'. It was the first time I'd felt that with any conviction. I gave him his bottle and he cried and drank, cried and drank. I thought he might have a pain. The nurse thought he was hungry but rebelling against the feed he was being given.

A few days later we were told he was being tried on different flavoured bottles. The nurses laughed, saying he had got his own way by kicking up so much about the feed. He got chocolate-flavoured one day and strawberry another but it only lasted three or four days, poor James. His output at the other end went up too much and he had to go back on a blander feed.

A few nights later I hit another crisis in myself – over-tired, I suppose. I lay awake crying, with everything going round and round in my head: my guilty ambivalence towards James, wishing he would die, not feeling really well myself any of the time, thinking I might as well get sterilised now and be done with it, wondering if Rick still loved me, worried that Stephen might be a coeliac and uncertain I took care of him well enough or even loved him enough. It was a real late-night, everything-out-of-proportion orgy of self-pity but fairly typical of how I felt still. I fell asleep eventually but, as always after a crying session, I woke up the next morning feeling woozy and distant. I resented going in to work but at least it distracted me.

Our schedule was still really punishing, with Rick working full-time office hours and me on shifts, having a one-year-old at home and a baby in the hospital, with all the washing needed for both, never mind having to to juggle the visits, the shopping and Stephen. On the days I worked four to midnight I had time with Stephen but not Rick, and I no longer had the luxury of coming home at teatime because that was when I went to the hospital.

Rick still seemed to be bearing up remarkably well but I knew he was very tired. It came out when he decided to go away for his weekend break. He was going to drive to a hotel in Connemara but before he left Dublin he went up to see James. He said James had been smiling at him and was really alert; his weight was up slightly. All combined to give Rick a good send-off. The feeds were now up to 45 ml a bottle – roughly the equivalent of an egg-cupful. But even before Rick left Dublin he said he began to feel slightly unwell and by the time he got to Connemara he was running a high temperature. It was as if even the sniff of relaxation, of switching off, was enough to knock him for six. He spent a good deal of the weekend in bed.

May continued to be a good month for James although we knew from the nurses that there was a certain amount of concern about his being on the TPN drip for so long and the fact that he still didn't seem capable of getting enough nutrition from his bottle feeds to put on weight. When it came to oral feeds more still seemed to be coming out than had gone in in the first place.

On the last Friday in May his white blood-cell count was up again, indicating yet another infection. There was also talk about putting in what's called a 'mainline' drip – this would be a semi-permanent site for the TPN. Every few days, sometimes even every day, the drip site was being changed so the poor little thing was like a pincushion from all the different veins that had been used. Sometimes the drip would be from one of his hands or, occasionally, one of his legs. His head was a good source of veins so it was often used but having a needle from your head is awkward. There are nurses in the hospital whose speciality is setting up drip-sites for babies and children but even they were finding James's little veins difficult. The drip site had had to be changed so many times. Sometimes we would find that the drip had come out and, in the period before the nurse should insert a new one, heaps of blankets would be put over James to heat him up because when you're warm your veins show more. Occasionally the drip's coming out was a bonus for us because it meant he could be put in the pram well covered with blankets and taken for a walk around the hospital. This was a big treat – you could always see it in his eyes. He seemed to take in every scrap of colour and shape, almost dazzled by this other world outside his room in Special Care.

The insertion of the mainline drip, however, while it would be easier on James physically, required a small operation. That meant an anaesthetic so we were a bit apprehensive.

Despite the nurses' constant encouragement and good-humoured banter about James's knowing that his Mum had arrived and their reassurance that I was giving him just what he wanted, a good cuddle, I was never really sure that he knew me at all. However, one Saturday afternoon one of the nurses who specialised in changing drip sites called up to his room while I was there and went straight over to James to say hello. He took one look at her and immediately began to cry loudly and convincingly. She turned to me and said it was awful, that none of the children liked them because they knew what was in store when they saw them coming. I just could not get over James's reaction. I was convinced from that small incident that, if he could distinguish that nurse from all the others, then he must know me too.

My sister later described a similar incident when she visited James with Rick. When they arrived James seemed to be dozing; at any rate his eyes were closed. Rick just said, 'Hello James,' and it was amazing how he immediately opened his eyes to see his dad. She was sure that he had recognised his voice.

James himself, though, never made any attempt to coo or gurgle or try out his voice in any way. He had a very expressive face but no repertoire of sounds. I noticed that he was not the only silent baby either. One of the other long-term babies was exactly the same.

In the last weekend in May Rick's mother and youngest sister, Marie Therese, arrived for a week's visit. Unfortunately James was back on antibiotics and rather tired but Mrs Boyle could still see a huge difference in him compared with three months previously. It was Marie Therese's first chance to meet James and I was glad she saw him at that stage. It was also nice for us, introducing him to someone new. We got so few chances to introduce him to anyone and, despite all the mixed feelings, I did feel good 'showing him off' to his aunt and grandmother.

The week they were with us went by quickly. Luckily James's infection was not nearly as bad as at Easter and the antibiotics cleared it up. It was also the week of my birthday and that evening, when I was in with James he was all smiles at me, almost as if he knew!

As I was leaving the hospital I met the registrar. He was with someone else but stopped me briefly to tell me that James had developed a hernia. He said it wasn't a serious problem and explained it in terms of a balloon pushing out and needing to be pushed back in. Although it was another problem it didn't upset me nearly as much as the feet episode and I felt, from my brief conversation with the registrar, that it was not too serious.

The following day Mrs Boyle and Marie Therese went home. We all called to see James before going out to the airport and he was in good form. When we brought Stephen in to see his little brother he pointed at James and said 'baby' – another first!

At the airport I met a friend of a friend with his wife, little girl and new baby boy. We got talking and I told them, briefly, about James. They told me their daughter had a rare pathological syndrome and was mentally handicapped. They told us she'd had fifteen operations so far. Her condition hadn't been properly diagnosed until she was a year old, and then only because they had kept insisting there was something wrong with her. She was now four and they said the last year hadn't been so bad, that it took ages to accept but that you do eventually. It was a relief to talk to someone who had some idea of what we were going through ourselves.

Rick's eldest sister, Anne Marie, had sent us a book about Great Ormond Street Hospital in London. It was called *Children First and Always*, which is the hospital's motto. I had great expectations when I began reading it, hoping to find someone I could identify with, some other mother as ambivalent as I was, some child as rare as our James. I felt bitterly disappointed as I read on and also angrier than ever. All the parents in the book seemed to me such selflessly devoted people that I couldn't possibly hope to emulate any of them. Most of their children had been planned and all the parents seemed to accept their children's diseases and deformities and desperately want them to live at all costs. Most of the mothers didn't work or else gave up their jobs because of the child. Only two of the children, in my judgement, were physically worse off than James. One of them was paralysed from the neck down, the other had such a list of problems which persisted over years that her parents' marriage broke up under the strain. Yet her mother continued to care for her devotedly.

We were now heading towards the middle of June, the longest summer evenings. James's weight was up again and the medical team was trying gradually to reduce the amount of TPN he was getting and to increase his bottle feeds. He got a bad dose of thrush, which made him cross but was treatable. His birth certificate arrived and it was correct – a male, named James Francis. It was something to hold on to, like a proof. The day after it arrived I was once again wishing James had never been born, wishing I was sterile, back to taking it all out on God, feeling I hated him, feeling that, if he was all he was cracked up to be that he would understand how I felt. I realised that I could never again believe in the God of my the childhood; that benevolent being who had watched over and cared about my every move all day and all night had deserted me for ever.

On 19 June I ran again in the women's Mini Marathon. I had done all of them up to then and when I met a running friend of long standing about six weeks beforehand she had vigorously encouraged me to get sponsorship for Crumlin Hospital. I'd been hesitating, partly from lack of energy, and saying I might do that the following year but she said no, this was the year our baby was there. She said she would start me off by sponsoring me herself. So, in the face of that enthusiasm I did collect money from people at work and the family. One of the nurses was also training for it and so we used to compare notes in the lead-up. It was getting to the stage that we knew more about the nurses' lives than the lives of our friends because the hospital was almost our only social life. The nurses seemed to have adopted James. Even those who weren't minding him knew him well and would pop in to say hello to him and to another baby boy in the same room as he who had been in

Special Care for about the same length of time. I used to feel sometimes that he had about twenty mothers.

For the previous few years we had tried, Denise and I, to make sure that my father got some kind of a short holiday every year. He said Rick and I had too much on our plates already to look after my mother so he arranged with the public health nurse, who came to give her a bath when she could, that she would go into Baggot Street Hospital for two weeks 'respite care' as it's called. She went in the day after the Marathon. I packed her case and saw her off and then went in to see her with my father before I started work at four o'clock.

Neither of us was terribly happy with the situation and, for the first week, my father seemed to spend as much time and effort going in to visit her as he usually did looking after her at home. That first afternoon I felt really fed up leaving her. Then on my tea break I went up to visit James and thought how true it was that a children's hospital, no matter how awful the illnesses, is nonetheless always a place full of hope, whereas old people who are ill often don't even have the hope that things could improve.

Despite all my mixed-up feelings and the agonising I went through every day I used to be remarkably calm and sure while I was actually holding James in my arms. It was as if his presence calmed me down and made things easier. It was during all the other hours of the days and nights, when I was so far away from him, that the dark thoughts, imaginings and endless speculating got the better of me.

I got the chance to bring two other friends in to see James on separate occasions. The first, whom I'd been friendly with for the best part of twenty years, is probably the only true atheist that I know. She's both very realistic and sympathetic and she had asked if she could meet James. It was nice, the few times it happened, to have a companion.

The second friend was Ciaran, who was home from Rome. He drove me to the hospital, which was the most wonderful relaxing treat. Ciaran's spontaneous reaction when he saw James was that he looked really well. He certainly did have a beautiful little face and big grey eyes. It was nice to see someone so enthusiastic but I knew as well that it was unrealistic because you couldn't judge how James was just by his face. He could look so cute, all dressed up in little outfits with none of his problems visible. When the nurse said she was going to change James's nappy Ciaran said he'd wait outside.

As June ended Rick and I were both struggling with chronic exhaustion. I remember one social event where both of us just felt as if we'd arrived from another planet. It was so difficult to make small talk and appear normal that I just couldn't wait to get away from it.

The doctor was still struggling with James's TPN levels and desperately trying to reduce them. One day she insisted that James must wear a cap or hat so as not to lose any heat, meaning energy, from his head. One of the nurses passed this information on to me and I brought in a little blue, knitted helmet which buttoned under his chin and a sailor's hat which the nurses thought was gorgeous on him but kept slipping down over his eyes. I felt the poor doctor must really be finding his nutrition maintenance a terrible challenge when she'd become so insistent about the hat.

Often now the nurses put James in his baby bouncer, either up in the cot or down on the floor. Rick and I spent hours each trying to teach him to grasp a rattle or toy until eventually he succeeded, even if he was then inclined to forget he was holding something and hit himself with it. We made the red elephant play its tune for him, because it caught his eye still.

We had asked Ciaran about having James christened. Although he had been baptised the night he was born he could still have a christening ceremony and we really wanted that. I felt that, if he was going to grow up, we should have a special day for him with photographs to remind him of it. The hospital chaplain willingly permitted it to be held in the chapel and Ciaran said he would do the ceremony. We had asked Rick's eldest sister, Anne Marie, to be godmother. She had several god-daughters already but this was her first godson. She was planning to come over to visit us from Germany at the end of July so that seemed a good time to have it but the complicating factor was that now the doctors were talking about James's second operation. A different surgeon was to be the man in charge of this huge undertaking – an attempt to close James's bladder.

The second big operation, which once again was to have a fifty-fifty chance of success, had never completely left the picture but it hadn't seemed imminent at any stage. It had been spoken of more in terms of towards the end of James's first year. Now consultations were taking place about how exactly it could be done and July or August were being mentioned.

One afternoon when I was visiting, the surgeon from the first operation was doing his rounds. It was a long time since I had seen him. He simply said that our baby was quite stable now after a very rocky patch; a very rocky patch, he repeated, emphasising his words.

We arranged the christening provisionally for the last Saturday in July as Anne Marie would be with us then, and Denise and Ken would be over. The operation now seemed to be pencilled in for August.

Before either of these momentous events, however, James had another big adventure: we were told we could arrange to take him home for the day. We were both really excited at the prospect and said we would take him home the following Sunday. He was now off the TPN drip for several hours a day, which made the trip possible.

James now weighed 3.71 kilos or about eight pounds. While I was in with him the day before the nurse, one of those who often minded him now, showed me how to change the dressing for his colostomy bag. She was so used to doing it herself she could have done it in her sleep but because she had to show me which bits were to be stuck together she got mixed up and stuck the two sticky sides, making both of us laugh over it. With the next demonstration she got it right and I too got the hang of it but I couldn't help hoping I wouldn't need to change it when he was home. I knew I'd be nervous doing it. Still, I was really looking forward to the next day. We said we would be in before twelve to collect him. In the meantime we kept our fingers crossed that James wouldn't develop a complication like a temperature overnight.

Margaret, yet again, minded Stephen the following morning while Rick and I went to the hospital to collect James. The Moses basket that Stephen had had was across the back seat of the car, waiting for James. When we got in to Special Care he was already off the drip but there were still a few things to be done and it was about half an hour later before he was finally put into my arms and we had the all-clear to leave.

The proud parents walked down the stairs together, and Rick said he would bring the car right up to the door so I waited just inside. I felt really emotional, standing there with James in my arms. For the very first time since he was born I felt he was mine – really and truly mine. There was no one to tell me what to do or not to do – I could hold him and look after him by myself just for these few hours. He was only on loan to us for five hours but we would all be together as a family in our own house for the first time. January seemed so very long ago. I still couldn't help thinking of what might have been – the ritual at the Coombe as the nurse carries your baby out to the car and hands your baby over to your custody at just five days old. Instead, here I was ten days short of six months later, borrowing my baby on a strict curfew arrangement.

It was a wonderful day and everything went better than we could have hoped for. Margaret and Don came down to our house for a little while and my parents also came up and we all took turns holding James, who seemed to enjoy every minute of the attention, smiling at everyone as well as looking around at all the new sights. Then everyone went home and we had time together. Stephen, too, was able to see James in a normal environment for the first time and reached over to touch 'baby' every so often. James was a model baby – he took his bottle well. I managed to change his nappy but left the colostomy bag alone. He slept for about an hour and a half in the basket; we peeped in at him every so often. Apart from the site for his drip, which was in his right arm that day and so was held firm in a splint, he looked like any normal baby.

Those few hours did me so much good it's almost impossible to describe the transformation. Even standing inside the door of Crumlin, before we left I felt, for the first time, that I really loved James and that I so wanted to bring him home and that, yes, I would do anything to have him home, that we would manage somehow. It was like a wonderful release to be able to feel that after such a long time.

Having James at home also boosted our confidence. It might only be a few hours but we managed well – not just managed: we all enjoyed ourselves, including James. I felt we'd been able to give him a special day even if he never remembered it. Rick took photographs too.

Rick had said he would take James back to Crumlin and that was what I wanted. I didn't really want to have to hand him back so I gave Rick the tough job because I felt he'd be better able for it than me. I stayed at home with Stephen. That evening, as after any special occasion, there was the let-down of its being all over. Once again James was ten miles away being minded by nurses and the few hours in our house had just gone by in a flash. But I will always be grateful to the enlightened doctor who had seen how important it was for all of us that James be allowed to visit his home and who had managed to get him to a stage where it became possible.

But by Wednesday James had another infection and his doctor told us that she would be turning up the drip again when he was over it. That wasn't good news. We knew there was concern about his being on TPN for so long but he still wasn't absorbing oral feeds sufficiently to be able to survive on them alone.

I still sometimes thought of the Catholic Church's position that one shouldn't use 'extraordinary means' to keep someone alive and wondered how they would define that stance exactly. Once again it's the double-edged sword of modern medicine. As the surgeon had told us in those first few days, it's very hard to die nowadays. The obverse of that is that people's faith in modern medicine is so great they sometimes take it to mean that it must be possible to save every life – and that's especially understandable when their own child is involved. They feel they should move mountains, go to America or London, raise half a million pounds or whatever it takes to save that life. The truth is that it still isn't possible to save every life and I still believe there are lives, including children's lives, where a decision eventually has to be taken that less intervention rather than more is the right path. That isn't easy on anyone – doctors or nurses, never mind parents – but in the end medicine can only go so far and then nature or God or fate or whatever you will has its way.

James's birth and short life to date had called into question everything that before I had felt was firm: my own faith in God, what makes us male and female, men or women, my own feelings and instincts, my own identity and what my life was about. Nothing was certain any longer and I had to learn to live with the uncertainty.

It's not at all nice to feel you're rejecting your own baby, which was what I had felt deep inside all along. But feelings are not something you can change overnight. You can do all in your power to carry out your duties and responsibilities and that may salvage something. Eventually it may even nourish a love over time but with a severely handicapped child there are so many aspects in the complicated equation of care and needs and allocation of time that there isn't always the luxury of sorting it all out. Mixed feelings are inevitable at some stage. The mothers who can keep their positive feelings to the fore are, I now believe, lucky, but not necessarily better, than the mothers who are overwhelmed by the negative. Even with a hundred-per-cent unequivocal love a child with extra, special needs puts greater responsibilities on a mother's shoulders and requires more of her than any single person can at all times provide.

Undoubtedly there are hundreds and hundreds of wonderful mothers who are to be greatly admired for their efforts in caring for their special children. It is, however, too easy and too pat simply to praise them for being wonderful; no one becomes a wonderful person easily or quickly and that attitude makes it all too easy to ignore the mothers who have greater difficulties in coping with their children and who may fester away for years with a painful mixture of conflicting emotions, a sense of failure or resentment and, worst of all, a terrible sense of guilt.

I really do think every mother who has a disabled child should be given at least one counselling session with a professional. They may never need another but it could prevent so much guilt and confusion just to be told by someone outside the family that they are normal, that their confusion is normal, that they are not alone in their feelings. Even to be warned that they may have these feelings and not to be taken by surprise by them would be salutory. I know I could have done with some such help. Although I muddled on it took me, I'd say, until about two years after James's death to be able to see the situation with any kind of perspective or even to give myself permission to mourn him. Up until then I felt I had no right to mourn – that that was Rick's sole prerogative, because I had wanted him to die and he had died and I had got my wish.

I know I've referred only to mothers in the previous paragraphs. That's deliberate because I can't speak for fathers. I only know that the relationship between a mother and her baby is different because of the physical connection between the two. This makes for a most intimate relationship when the relationship works. I think the very intimacy of the bond, however, compounds the difficulties when, for whatever reason, the relationship does not work. There aren't quite the same expectations of fathers.

That month of July it certainly wasn't true that I constantly wanted James to die. I still thought often that it would be best for him if he did not live beyond childhood but even then I was beginning to be able to see a future for him, even if only a short future. I still hadn't got to grips with the problems he was likely to have as an older child, much less an adolescent or an adult. The reels of mental pictures of his future went on rolling around my brain night and day, but I could just about see my way to two or three years ahead. I also had to consider the awful grief that the loss of a brother at that stage would mean for Stephen.

On the whole, though, July was the best month of the summer, in fact of the whole year. I was less agitated, somehow. I really began to learn to live each day as it came. Whenever my mind started the usual whine: 'But what will you do when he comes home? How will you manage then?' I would just shut it with the thought: he may never come home and if he does we'll deal with it then. When I thought: how long can you go on like this, working, and minding Stephen and visiting the hospital? I would try to squash that fear too by telling myself that I could only keep going a day at a time for as long as I could. However bad the thought, there was always the reassurance that it might never happen.

James's visit home was a huge morale boost. It helped me to let go and really love this helpless, beautiful baby of ours and that, in turn, meant I hated myself less. Of course there were still bad days and terrible, haunting doubts but for a while they were less acute. James seemed to be spewing up bits of his feeds quite a lot but that might have been caused by the infection. When he was finished that course of antibiotics the drip was turned up again and he started to put on weight. By 20 July he was over four kilos for the first time. The scale read 4.09 kilos and by the following day 4.19 kilos.

That day we took Stephen to the zoo for the first time. Margaret and Don and their little girl came too. We all wanted to see their reactions to the animals and it had taken a couple of weeks to organise an afternoon when we would all be free to go. It was sunny. Stephen thought everything was a bird because my parents had a bird and that was as near to anything 'wildlife' that he'd ever known. He also had his first ice cream cone that afternoon and thoroughly enjoyed it. Despite our best intentions that was the only organised outing of the summer but we still talk about it and tell Stephen about it. One Saturday afternoon, soon afterwards, Rick brought home a beautiful fire engine on wheels which Stephen could sit on. It was a dream toy for a little boy and is driven around our house to this day.

The morning after the zoo we had an appointment with the registrar to discuss James and the plans for the next operation. We were up at a quarter to seven to get to the hospital by a quarter to eight so that we could see him before he began his daily rounds. He described the operation to us: an attempt would be made to close the bladder so as not have it open to the air. He said an orthopaedic surgeon would also be involved as they would need to break some bones in the hip area and reset them. I found that part upsetting. He was optimistic overall, but then he always was optimistic about James. He used to tell us he would be able to play rugby when he was older. He also said without being too specific that there could be possible problems and difficulties. We had brought Stephen with us and we all stood around James's cot, talking about this big operation while he was oblivious to what was planned for him.

I was extra tired, from the previous day's outing, the early start and the tension associated with any consultation about James. That meant I also felt depressed again; the two went hand-in-hand. I used to look in the mirror and think I looked so awful it somehow justified my feeling depressed. I was only about seven and a half stone at that stage. Even though I attempted three meals a day I often hardly tasted the food or was too tense to enjoy it because I'd be rushing to the hospital or to catch the bus to work. In general I felt I was not the same person I had been a year before: I felt much older and sadder. Sometimes I felt so tired I wished my own life was over just so that I could have a long rest.

One Monday I took Stephen in with me to James. Luckily James was off the drip so I was able to take them both out to the ward corridor, wheeling Stephen in the buggy while I held James in the crook of one arm and made animal noises for both of them, showing them the pictures of different animals on a poster on the wall. The nurses laughed at me, saying I really had my hands full.

The following evening Rick's oldest sister, Anne Marie, arrived off the boat. On the Wednesday I brought Anne to meet James for the first time and to introduce him to his godmother. We sat by his cot for a full hour and a quarter and he just slept and slept but Anne kept telling me not to disturb him. I think she was quite happy just admiring him for the time being. At last he stirred and woke up smiling at us and you couldn't but be captivated by him.

The next day James had an infection and although he was a bit better by the following day he wasn't feeding well. We were very nervous about the christening the next day, hoping it wouldn't have to be postponed. We had invited about a dozen friends and Denise and Ken were coming for the weekend as well as my parents and Anne.

On the thirtieth of July James was christened by Ciaran in the chapel of Crumlin Hospital. It seemed a big achievement to have got him that far. For the first time our friends were able to see him and everyone made a big effort for us. Anne and I had gone into the hospital very early to get James dressed but by the time all the nursing jobs had been completed we only had about ten minutes left. Still, he was ready in time and looked beautiful. Anne had bought Stephen a new outfit of a green T-shirt and shorts the previous day and he looked splendid with a little navy cardigan and his sheen of golden hair. After the christening, of course, we had to leave James back up to the ward and say goodbye to him for a while but we left him in the christening robe. We had also bought a cake which said: 'For all my nurses, love James'.

We brought everyone to a local pub for coffee and sandwiches and cake. We had decided not to have anything at home – partly because it was too far away from the hospital, but more because James's absence would be too hard to take in our own house. It's not easy to have a christening party without a baby. His absence seemed just that bit less obvious in the pub.

In the afternoon we were able to leave Stephen with Anne and Denise while we went back in to see James again, not liking to leave him alone on his big day. Rick fed him his bottle but unfortunately he threw it all back up. Luckily Rick had been using a big terry nappy as bib and it took most of it. After that we changed him out of his finery and back into ordinary baby clothes.

Rick collected the christening photos and some of them were just beautiful. I was even more glad that we had made it a special occasion.

The following afternoon Anne and I took Stephen in with us to James. It was still much easier bringing him with a second adult. James was very alert and drank two thirds of his bottle. He weighed 4.53 kilos or nearly ten pounds. The nurse told us they had stopped putting cornflour in his bottle and that the next plan was to turn off his drip between six and eight in the morning to see if that would increase his appetite.

On the Thursday morning Anne went back to England. James's operation had been provisionally set for 22 August and, although we knew that could change, the same date had been consistently mentioned for some time now. With Anne gone it seemed to be looming very near, just two and half weeks away. James would be seven months old on the twenty first.

The first Sunday in August Rick and I went in to visit James together in the afternoon as I had to start work at four o'clock. The nurse told us that we could have taken him home that afternoon and we were both really disappointed that we hadn't known. It certainly hadn't been from lack of asking but, once again, communications had failed us somewhere along the line. All the same, James was off the drip, so we made the best of that freedom by taking him for a long walk and, because it was a sunny afternoon we went out on to the steps of the hospital and let him feel the fresh, warm air. As always when he was out of that room he was alert and looking all around him.

A mother we'd got to know arrived while we were there and stopped to talk to us. She really didn't know any of the details about James's problems and I thought, as we stood there, how normal James looked, nestled in Rick's arms, obviously intelligent, with a perfectly-formed head and face and all the required limbs, fingers and toes. And still it was so hard to tell people the real problems, things that most people wouldn't be able to dream up if they tried.

I decided to take some leave from work in order to spend extra time at the hospital during the couple of weeks before the next operation. A few days I left for the hospital at about eleven in the morning and stayed till half past four or so, which meant I got to feed James at least once, and usually twice, and could take him out in the ward pram for walks when he was off the drip. But even that time with him had to be stolen from Stephen so I didn't spend every day with him.

With just over a week to go before the operation we again got the chance to bring James home for the day. I went to collect James on my own so that Rick could be with Stephen. It was less momentous than on the first occasion but still terribly exciting. Again we had visitors, but also time on our own. James was a less than model baby this time too, and threw up a large part of his bottle so that he needed to be changed completely. Despite Stephen being below par, we managed to get both of them on the floor together while Stephen played with a toy and James looked on and I caught glimpses of a possible future with James at home.

Denise was over all that following week as part of her summer holidays. She had to leave again on the Friday night because she and Ken were going on to the Lake District. Rick and I had also arranged a week away, starting a week after the date of the operation. On the Friday afternoon Denise, Stephen and I once again visited James. He was taken off the drip and we were able to take him out for his ramble in the pram.

On our way out we met Sr Anna. She stopped for a short chat and warned me to expect James to be quite sick after the operation. She also said a certain number of setbacks were likely. It crossed my mind, during that conversation, how inappropriate it was for us to have arranged to go away to Connemara ourselves for a week's break so soon after the operation. However, in my new one-day-at-a-time-mode, I thought there was no point in cancelling at that stage. We could do so if we needed to. On we went in a posse and, in the distance, we saw James's surgeon from the first operation. Then we met the registrar, who stopped for a brief hello.

When we finally got back to the ward Denise said it was as if James's entire life had passed before him during that one walk because he'd met nearly all the people who had been most involved in his care. I wasn't too keen on the analogy as it seemed like a bad, rather than a good, omen.

If it was omens I was looking for the next day was worse. At work I got a bomb scare call which really shook me and I had to phone the gardai about it. I felt sick at the thought that it could be real and I know I would have felt personally responsible if anything had gone off in Dublin that day. Rick, in the meantime, was in at the hospital and called for me on his way home. He said there had been an emergency in James's room while he was there and that an operation had had to be performed in the room. The child was out of danger by the time he left but Rick was obviously badly affected by it. We were both shaken and tired that night.

The following day was Sunday, the day before James's second operation. Rick and I had asked my father to babysit for us as we had decided to go in to see James late, after Stephen was in bed. That way we would see him as near as possible to this operation.

It was a near-perfect visit. James was awake and the nurse was joking about how he was going to manage through the night without his feeds as he had to fast from midnight. The registrar, who never really seemed to go off duty, came up to see us too and the three of us stood around James's cot while he looked from one face to the other as if he was wondering what he had done to deserve to have all his favourite people with him together that evening. I'm so glad he could not anticipate what was ahead.

When the registrar had left we stayed on together for a while, until eventually James drifted off to sleep.

11

SECOND OPERATION

James's second operation was six and a half hours long. He had left the ward by the time we rang at a quarter to nine that morning. 'Just left,' we were told. It was to be a long, long wait. Rick phoned at eleven o'clock and was told the operation was going to take longer than expected and that James would definitely be going to intensive care afterwards. That was the first blow of the day. That sinking feeling. Nerves heightened. We asked Margaret down for coffee and a chat, desperately making conversation to help pass the time.

At lunchtime I suggested we go into the hospital as I felt I couldn't bear to wait at home any longer. Rick wondered what would be the point. I just wanted to be there. I felt it would be easier to pass the time somehow. We left at one o'clock. We were in the hospital by a quarter to two. Rick had had the foresight to bring plenty of change in case we needed to phone. We went up to Special Care. It was a bit of a shock to see another baby there, in James's place, as if he'd never been there.

The staff nurse told us James was still in theatre but that she'd go and ask how things were going. Another hour at least, we were told. She took us up to the intensive care waiting-room. The door was locked but another couple was waiting inside. The nurse had to go and get a key. I felt impatient waiting outside although I had absolutely no reason to be in a rush. I couldn't hurry up the operation. The couple inside hadn't realised they'd been locked in. The nurse left the door slightly open so that it wouldn't happen again. The wife and I began talking. Their six-year-old boy had just had a heart operation but was said to be recovering well in Intensive Care. They told us they'd been in to see him twice and he'd recognised them and said hello but that he was not yet out of the anaesthetic. They were just waiting to see the surgeon. They had one other child, an older girl, who was at home with her granny. The wife seemed quite nervous and smoked. The father was a genial man, quite eager to chat. Getting some of the anxiety out of his system, I suppose.

They asked us about James. We told them he was having an operation on his bladder. They couldn't know how serious that was. People don't generally hear of operations on babies' bladders. Hearts, yes; kidneys, yes; even lungs, but not bladders. We were on our own in that regard. Time passed. The couple told us they'd booked into the parents' wing for the week and they praised it, saying it was very reasonable and that there were showers and a kitchen. They said they didn't know Dublin well.

The ICU waiting-room was less severe, less disinfected than most other parts of the hospital. It had a carpet, a net curtain on the glass door to the corridor, curtains on the outside window – a vestige of privacy. There were two armchairs and a long settee, a coffee table with a tiled top. On it were a small pile of leaflets about ICU, telling parents to make their visits brief but frequent. It explained some of the terminology you might hear: respirator, transfusion, and so on.

On the walls of the room were photos of the work of ICU – nurses lifting babies, machines, wires. The photos looked slightly dated, their colour a bit washed out. Other photos were of hopes realised – children who'd been in ICU going home, making their First Communion six months later.

The window was open and the curtains were blowing slightly in the draught from the door but it was hot and stuffy in that room. The father got up and went in to see his son again. He came back. The boy had said hello again but was going back to sleep.

I suggested to Rick that we ask about James again. He was told that James was still in theatre but was expected to be out in about half an hour. It was nearly three o'clock. I thought of his tiny body laid out on an operating table for all this time, surrounded by surgeons, nurses, anaesthetist, and having God knows what done to him.

Another woman came into the room. She was crying. She sat down and seemed noisy in the silence. She began apologising for crying. The other mother asked her if everything was all right. She said her son was going to be all right but that he had a tube down him and they were waiting for it to be taken out. He was retching and really crying and she just couldn't watch him any more; she'd had to come out. She said her boy had been in ICU since the previous Monday but was going to be moved to another ward that day. After a while she calmed down. She asked the other couple how their boy was getting on, asked us had we a child in theatre. We told her. Seven months old. The bladder. Told her he'd been down there since nine o'clock that morning.

She told us about another boy who'd been in theatre for seven hours the previous Monday. She said it was only the second time in the world that particular operation had been carried out and the first time in Ireland. She said his heart had stopped eleven times since then but that now he was starting to come on. Imagine, eleven times, she said, after that she'd never give up hope. 'You just can't. You have to keep praying.

Another young woman came in but backed out when she saw

the room was quite full. The man jumped up to give her his seat but she said she'd wait outside; she'd rather really! When asked if her daughter was still down there she just said she was. She went back out on to the landing to sit, to pace, to watch, to wait.

I was feeling more and more tense. The wait seemed to have been so very long then; since that morning, since the previous night, since January. Staring out through the window panes at oblong patches of grey sky, the curtains shifting slightly, the photos on the walls, our hands. We couldn't say a lot at that stage. The other mother went out for a smoke. I said I would go out and ask again.

Just past half past three I rang the bell outside the doors of ICU. A nurse came out after what seemed like ages. Rick had joined me. She told us James was out but they had to fix him up and 'take some bloods'. She told us he was 'very shook', that they would cover up as much as they could before we came in.

We walked slowly over to the bench on the landing and sat down. Half-relief rushed through us, swamping some of the fear. At least he was out; he had survived the operation. After a few minutes we wandered back into the waiting-room and sat down again. We told the other parents he was out, that we would be allowed in to see him as soon as they were ready.

We all waited again. The couple from the country couldn't see their son's surgeon until he was finished the last operation for that day. Time passed very slowly again. We looked at the ICU leaflet. Short, frequent visits, we read again. Say the things you normally say to your child; reassure him. That passed about two minutes.

I went and read the captions on the photos of children who had recovered, left ICU and Crumlin and gone home. Twenty minutes, maybe more, passed. I couldn't bear it any longer. They were taking a long time. I said I'd go and ask if we could go in yet. It's about fifteen metres from the waiting room to the outer door of ICU. The sister and I met halfway. She was a kindly woman, but also appraising, with a ready smile.

'I was just coming for you,' she said. 'Is your husband there?'

I rushed back to get Rick.

She told us James was not a good colour. No matter what they did or what she told us it was still going to be a shock when we saw him. She said he was quite grey and very tired. The necessary tubing had been put in place in case he needed to go on a ventilator. She advised us just to come in for a few moments to see him and then to come back again when we were ready.

We were still eager to see him, to see with our own eyes how he was, how he'd got through it. We were let in the doors to the small hallway. We washed our hands, put on aprons. There was dread too. We held hands tightly and walked in together.

James's face was quite altered. It was swollen; his eyes were shut and one of them seemed quite swollen too. His head was shaking, rolling from side to side with enormous, frantic energy. We couldn't see him from the waist down. He was covered with a little cotton sheet, a baby's cot sheet. His legs were bound together, as they'd warned us they would be, but they were also raised up and hooked onto something a bit like traction. It was as if the bottom half of him was crucified. We spoke to him, called him by name. His head was still rolling. He seemed to be in distress. We were told that might well be because he might be having some difficulty breathing. The sister said he might have to go on a ventilator if he wasn't getting enough oxygen.

He was greyish all right but it was his puffy face, his little suspended legs and his desperately rolling head that were more upsetting. After a couple of minutes we looked at each other, nodded and started to go back out. The sister told us we could come back in a while.

We went back out to the dark landing. I took a deep breath. We sat on the bench by the wall – just sat, assimilating what we'd seen. Looking back on it, I realise that was the last time we ever saw James even remotely look like the child we'd come to know, the last time we ever saw him breathing on his own.

The registrar came up the stairs. He saw us and came over. He gave us the impression that the operation had gone reasonably well but that he had reservations. He said they were concerned about the length of time it had taken and at the trauma that might have caused James. He said the tissue had not been 'at all friendly' and that they were not optimistic that the bladder would stay closed. So further surgery fairly soon seemed on the cards. But we had been warned of that.

At least James's operation was over. Nothing serious had gone wrong. The awful tension of the long wait had been broken but the picture of tiny James and his distorted face, of his legs tied together and the cot sheet covering what, presumably, was too awful to see – that was still very fresh. I kept saying I hoped they'd put him on a ventilator rather than leave him in distress.

We told Margaret by phone that the operation was over and had gone reasonably well: she and Don, too, were worried because it had taken so long. I asked her to collect Stephen from the babyminder's and said we should be home to put him to bed. She said she'd ring my father. We went back to our hard bench. I don't know how long afterwards it was that the registrar came back out to us.

'That son of yours,' he said in the tone of voice a teacher would use for a child needing a scolding. That was how he spoke of James, always, as if of someone he knew really well and cared about. But this was serious. He told us James was bleeding internally and that they had called the surgeon back in. He told us they would have to open James up again and try to stop the bleeding. I asked him if James had been put on a ventilator. He told us he had.

The fear and tension were back, heavier, tighter even than before. I suppose we were stunned.

How could James possibly take another operation, being opened up again when they had already told us he was exhausted? Rick was more optimistic than me, refusing to leap forward to the realm of possibilities. That had been the difference between us all along. He dealt with the here and now. I leapt into the future and all possible things that might, or might not, happen.

James's surgeon from the first operation came past a short time later and spotted us. He asked us how the surgery had gone. We told him things had just deteriorated and they had called the other surgeon back in because James was bleeding internally. He rushed in to see if he could do anything but was back in a couple of minutes. He said there was some bleeding but that things seemed under control and that that was what intensive care was for: dealing with situations like this. Another flicker of hope.

The other surgeon arrived and went straight in. We stayed sitting on the bench, holding hands. Soon he came back out and walked over to us. He spoke slowly: 'I'm afraid there's very little hope.' Rick broke down. It was a cry from his very depths. I knew in that moment how much he had hoped James would pull through and how much he loved him.

The surgeon grabbed our coats as I tried to hold Rick, to hug him. He said we didn't have to talk there. He told us to come inside. It was more private, he said. He guided us into the little waiting-room and closed the door. There was no one else in there. We sat down on the sofa. He sat in the far corner opposite us. He began talking again.

James was bleeding, not just from one or two places but, it seemed to him, from almost everywhere. He had had blood transfusions and they amounted to more than his own blood volume at this stage. Nothing had actually gone wrong during the operation but it had all taken longer than expected. By the time they had prepared him, then worked on the hernia, the bones . . . Then the tissue had been difficult. The length of time James had been on TPN was another factor against him. Although they had done an extremely good job of keeping up his nutrition and he was as good as he could possibly be, given his difficulties, there were still liable to be little deficiencies because the drip could never be as good, or provide nutrition as complete, as food assimilated normally. They had thought that his blood coagulation mechanism had broken down but the test had come back showing it was still functioning. He could open up James again but he was not hopeful of its being very successful.

In retrospect, I suppose he was also looking for our views in all this. I believe that if we had been vehemently against it, he would not have touched the tiny child again. But we had gone far past the non-intervention argument.

Rick said: 'Well we can only say what we've said all along: that we don't want you to push him too far. We want him to suffer as little as possible.'

The surgeon sat, his head hanging, his two hands dangling from his knees. He seemed tired. Really, we were leaving the decision to him.

Rick asked if James was not going to get better then how long would he be with us?

The reply was: 'Not long. Not long at all.'

After a long pause the surgeon got up and left us . . .

12

LITTLE HOPE

We had some phoning to do. I was glad that Rick had brought some change. We needed to call Margaret again and Rick said he had better ring his mum. When I got through I put my arms round him. He was shaky but was able to get the words out, to say they said there was very little hope. The other mother, who was still waiting for her daughter to return from theatre, was using the other phone. Someone else was waiting. I said I'd go down and ring Margaret from downstairs. I flew down. I felt I was in a huge rush although in fact I knew I wasn't – it was just the tension driving me, my whole system on full alert.

The only phone I could find was right beside the front door. I told Margaret that everything had changed again, that James would have to be opened up again, was bleeding internally. Would she ring my father again? She would. I ran back upstairs.

We began waiting on the bench again Frozen. Trying to come to terms with the possibility that things might be hopeless. On one level you're thinking probably faster than normal. On another you're not thinking at all. Trying hard not to. Numbed. Extra aware of everything around you, including irrelevant details. We kept waiting for a glimpse of James being brought from ICU to theatre again. He would have to come out through the heavy double doors and be wheeled into the lift.

Eventually I said to Rick that if anything was going to happen I wanted to see James again. Rick was not so sure. The lift doors opened again: another child moving into ICU. It was the other mother's little girl.

In the end, at the risk of being a nuisance, I rang the ICU bell again. It was the sister who once again came out to me. I told her if anything was going to happen I wanted to see him again. Nothing was going to happen she assured me, half-smiling. So there was hope again. Also confusion, with the surgeon's words so recent. She went on to say that his heartbeat had stayed quite steady through it all and they were just fixing him up. She told me there was a bit to be done yet but that as soon as that was done she'd call us in again.

So it was over. The second, brief, operation had been done in ICU. He was steady. I went to tell Rick. Things were marginally less hopeless. But now Rick was not convinced, still believing the surgeon. We didn't see him again that evening.

My mind whirled, at times feeling James's death would be for the best and also feeling that if he died it was going to take a terrible toll on Rick; then again thinking that if he pulled through it was going to be an even longer and more tortuous route back to where we'd been yesterday and the entire operation was now a failure and he would have go through it all again.

Inside ICU it all took such a long time. They did, though, call us in at last. To our eyes things were a lot different.

James was completely still. Not a twitch. His face was still swollen but half-covered by the ventilator which was doing the hard work of breathing for him. His legs were no longer up. He was lying down flat. By opening him up again they had had to undo all the bone setting and attempted closing of the bladder. We really were back to square one. Only the hernia remained fixed after all that surgery. There was a long road ahead even if James pulled through.

Several times, in different ways, we asked to be told that he was not suffering. They assured us he was not. We spoke his name. We told him we were there. We put our fingers through his hands. Held each other's hands. I have never seen so many drips and tubes attached to anyone. They were still giving him blood, the nurse almost constantly checking the rates and flows.

It was time to go out again. Sister came with us. She said we should go and get something to eat and gave us directions to the staff canteen. We went down there, obediently. We were among the last, but one of the nurses from Special Care was there with a couple of other nurses we didn't know. They told us in the canteen that we couldn't have a meal because we didn't have a ticket or note from one of the sisters, but we could have a snack. It seemed so ludicrous talking about rules about meals in our situation.

The nurse we knew talked across to us from her table: 'How is James?' she asked. 'I believe he's out of theatre.'

We told her there was very little hope.

'Ah now, you know James is a fighter,' she said. 'Sister just told us he was a very bad colour when he got back up but that's just the length of the operation.'

She obviously hadn't heard what we'd heard. She didn't know. We left it. And yet Sister had said nothing was going to happen.

We went back upstairs. We saw the other boy's parents several more times. They had spoken to his surgeon and the operation had gone fine. This was a hugely traumatic day for them. They had made all sorts of arrangements, weeks in advance, preparing themselves for this day and now they could almost relax. I felt we were such veterans of it all at this stage, old-timers almost in this hospital.

The next couple of hours passed. No real change. Then we

were told the second operation had succeeded in easing, but not stopping, the bleeding. The surgeon really was wonderfully skilful. We were allowed back in and met the night nurse who was to look after James for the next twelve hours. The sister went off duty, but not before asking us if we wanted to stay the night in the hospital. She told us they could try to arrange for beds in the parents' wing. We got some change and phoned Margaret again to ask her if it would be all right. She said not to worry, she would of course look after Stephen. Later we were told they could get us single rooms only but that we could stay together in the ICU waiting-room if we liked. The sofa in there pulled out into a bed.

We went in to see James again. I don't think I saw him once in Intensive Care after that operation without crying. It was really upsetting just to look at him. So tiny, so ill, yet swollen, and now so motionless, attached to so many drips and the ventilator; with half his insides held together only by bandages and pads, as I visualised it, soaking up his blood.

The nurse was visibly affected also. She told us things were pretty critical, that she'd called for the doctor. He seemed very young. After examining James he told us nothing would happen before tomorrow evening. Another contradiction, it seemed. Yet the nurse, without contradicting him at all, seemed to give us a different message. She said, quite firmly, that she wanted one of us to stay in the hospital anyway − to stay the night, in case they had to call us. James was still very critical she said. Yes, the bleeding had eased but it had not stopped. Someone said they would get us tea. Where would we be? We would be in the waiting-room. We agreed again to stay together, nearby. It was late now, completely dark outside. I felt exhausted.

There was no one in the waiting-room now but us. The other parents, who were from outside Dublin, had all booked rooms in advance, once they'd known the date of their child's operation. The tea came. Rick said he'd like some bread. I said I'd get it for him from the parents' wing. I couldn't find it and had to come back upstairs and get directions from a nurse. I had to walk through the corridor of one of the other wards to get to it. It was all quiet and dark there, with two or three sleeping children in each room, it seemed. Sick children, but healthy compared with the ones upstairs in ICU and Special Care. I found the wing this time. Light was coming from the kitchen and the door was open. It was more relaxed in there than upstairs in the waiting-room, almost as if the parents were off duty. The parents we'd met earlier were there, drinking tea, much less tense than they had been in the afternoon, as well as a couple of people I hadn't met before. There was actually laughter as I came in but they were immediately solicitous. Of course I could have some bread, they told me. I took two slices and was given margarine. They asked how James was. I said he was still critical and that they wanted us to stay the night. They said encouraging things and I left quickly. The tea had been brought by the time I got back. We drank it. Rick ate the bread. There was nothing else to do then but go to bed.

I remember us settling down on that bed pulled out from the couch. Shoes off, clothes still on. I felt I was really overdosing on that waiting-room. The curtains were blowing slightly. We were composed. Things were very bad; yet this was what I had wanted, asked for, begged God for. I was getting my wish, it seemed. Every so often I asked myself the accusing question 'Now are you satisfied?' Yet the alternative seemed almost too much to contemplate at that juncture: the difficult struggle from near-death to another, perhaps more precarious, equilibrium. The same major operation all over again.

I know I fell asleep almost immediately. I'll always remember how, when I woke a couple of hours later, Rick said, almost accusingly, 'You fell asleep.' After that, rest was fitful. Even though we were lying down for something like six hours it was a long night. At one stage I remember Rick standing over at the window in the dark.

I got up before half past six, wide awake, all sleep gone. I rang the bell and went in to see James again. He lay so still. The nurse touched him gently, lovingly. She was almost constantly checking the drips, monitoring him. She told me he was much the same, still critical. She said she was sorry; she couldn't give us any more hope.

'He wasn't expected to last the night, you know,' she said. 'I was just told to keep him as comfortable as possible.'

It was back to the waiting-room. Later, I went down to the parents' corridor again, just to use the toilet and wash my face. The mother of the little boy who'd been due to move back down to a ward was just getting out of the shower. She asked how things were.

'Well, he's still alive,' I said.

'While there's life there's hope. Honestly. After seeing that other boy this week I believe anything's possible. I'll say a prayer for him.'

I asked about her boy. He had been moved down to a ward and was doing fine.

I went back up to the waiting-room.

Rick and I went to see James again. The night nurse was going off duty soon. She had no more to tell us. We would have to see what the doctors said when they came round. But we could see for ourselves too, watching James, listening to her.

Soon after the sister came on duty she came out to speak to us in the waiting-room. I think she said she was sorry. It was not the same message as the previous afternoon at all, when she had retained a certain optimism. She told us James had stopped producing urine and that really there was no point in giving us hope. I asked her about the previous night – how she had been so positive when everyone else was not. She said she was an eternal optimist and that, because she had seen so many terribly ill children who were not expected to make it, turning round and doing just that, she was always very slow to give up on them. Her face was kind and a little sad.

The surgeon came to speak to us also. He told us James could live for days. That was the hardest blow of that morning: the combination of hopelessness and the prospect of a slow death was hard to take. That, with all hope gone, we might still have a long, long wait of watching James so ill, so still, so unlike the bright-eyed baby we'd said goodnight to on Sunday night.

The sister told us we should take a break ourselves: go home for a while and maybe rest. She said they would phone us if anything at all happened. She asked about our other little fellow, hadn't we another child at home? We told her a neighbour was minding him. We were very tired.

Our old friend the registrar came in to us, briefly. 'I'm very sorry,' was what he said to us. He didn't stay long. Always on the move. But he was genuinely sad. He had, after all, been one of James's best friends. He knew James better even than most members of our own families. He'd been his advocate, I felt. He'd arranged his operation. He'd explained things to us. He had really believed James would grow up, despite his bags and incontinence problems, to play rugby. And now he too was telling us that he knew James wasn't going to make it.

We were almost too tired to make decisions and arrangements for another day, but we had to. We decided to go home together, as James's condition seemed unlikely to change much in the next few hours, and then to take turns coming back, especially if there were going to be more days of this intense watching and waiting. I think both of us found the thought of more days hard to face. The previous evening it had seemed that things would go either way very quickly. It was terribly upsetting to visit James and watch him and it was even harder now knowing we would just be watching his slow death.

We went in to see him once more. The day nurse had taken over his care. Tears started coming out of my eyes almost as soon as I reached his place each time. He didn't move at all. We would put one finger into his tiny, inert fist but there was no reaction. The drugs were making him puffier too; the little pointy face and almost translucent skin were gone. The sister asked us about booking a room for that night. We said that one of us would stay.

I decided I would ring two close friends and ask them if they'd be willing to stay a couple of nights each in our house in case we were called in during the night. We decided that I'd stay at home for the rest of the day while Rick went back and that I would spend the night in the hospital.

We got to Margaret and Don's. They made us tea. Stephen was running around but wanted to have nothing to do with us. It was the first time I'd ever seen him like that. If I tried to catch him he squealed and squirmed and referred everything to Margaret or Don. He was punishing us, I suppose, for abandoning him.

However, when we got back to our house, he settled down immediately and was his cheerful, affectionate self. My father called up to see us. We had breakfast and more tea. Then we both had showers. I felt I couldn't really sleep so didn't go to lie down.

Perversely, I said there still might be hope. I was so very afraid of what would happen if James did turn the corner that I needed to face that remote possibility. The prospect of being asked to watch him and worry over him for weeks, perhaps months, seemed at that stage a harder prospect than the final end, than his death. For it all to be over; not to have to watch him lying there, being breathed for, pumped, drugged, swelling unrecognisably; not even to have to worry for the years ahead; to have that black burden of grief and anxiety taken away – that would be far easier for me. So I felt I must not presume on it. But that just brought me back into the same old mental cycle of wanting him to die or not wanting him to die. My inner voice was still accusing me, relentlessly, of just wanting him to die. This was what you wanted all along, and now you're getting your way. Are you happy now? How dare you cry now, this was what you begged God for! I had to admit to myself that this was what I had thought, still thought, was for the best. But it was all much more painful, too, than I had thought possible and I knew Rick was taking it terribly hard.

Since the previous evening I had been all too aware of how far apart our positions, philosophically and emotionally, were towards James. With Rick, there was none of this guarded, qualified love that I felt towards him There was no resentment at all in Rick. He loved this second child of his totally, without reservation, and he had really believed he would make it.

There was another important factor in the equation also. All through the past seven months Rick had done his absolute best to support me, when he hardly knew how to support himself. I had been on an emotional see-saw, up and down. Suffering, certainly, but needing someone strong to keep me on the tracks. Now I felt that in the space of twelve hours the tables had been turned and Rick needed my support more than I needed his. He was facing something terrible, the loss of a beautiful baby that he'd loved so much. I envied him the absolute purity of his emotions compared with my confused, and as I saw them, sullied ones.

There were more phone calls to be made, to be answered. Mary said she would come out to stay, several nights if necessary; we were not to worry about anything. When things are bad people do so much – and you ask things of them that you would never normally ask. One of the mothers I was friendly with from Special Care phoned to offer help as well. My father broached the question of a grave. He said if, as it now seemed possible, James was not going to be with us much longer, we should think about it. Would we like to use the grave in Kilmacanogue? My maternal grandmother is buried there. I assured Rick it was a really beautiful place, that graveyard, and he said that would be all right with him. My father said he would make enquiries. He also offered us the use of his car. He was anxious to do something to help us and kept telling us we should take some rest. I gladly took his car in case Rick was called in during the night.

It was a mainly quiet day of tiredness, time on our hands and James continuously on our minds but it was a relief to spend the hours with Stephen at home. Calls to the hospital brought news that there was no change. After lunch Rick set off again, with supplies of change for the call-box. He rang during the afternoon, full of praise for the nurse now with James. He also said Sr Anna wanted to see us.

Rick arrived home again before Stephen went to bed and the three of us had a short time together. Then it was time for me to go back.

After eight o'clock it was always quieter in the hospital, even in the main corridor that buzzed so much during the day. I went up the stairs. Past Special Care. If only I could have been back to the relative stability of Special Care that had become like home to us over the months. It *was* James's home. Up the second flight of stairs to ICU. I rang the bell, washed my hands, put on the apron, saw him and cried yet again. Even knowing what I was going to see couldn't prepare me for it. Each time it was just as hard; each time the tears came when I saw the pitiful little scrap of James's body, so broken, so unworkable, so perfect in so many parts. He was more swollen than he had been that morning. His skin seemed taut with it, especially his eyelids, wrists and fingers. I cried for myself and for the loss of the delicate little baby we had last seen on Sunday night: those fine, thin fingers, tiny-boned, the little pointed face and bright, bright grey-blue eyes. The swelling was horrible but if that was the price to be paid for keeping him out of pain then it had to be.

The night nurse was back on now, the same one as before. She asked me if I would like to hold James but she warned that holding him would involve a risk to his life, as they would have to take him off the ventilator for a second or so and switch to a manual pump while he was being moved. (The manual process was called 'bagging'.) I said I would like to but that if there was a risk then I couldn't do it without Rick's being there. I said I'd phone him. One of the nurses told me that if I wanted a bed to check in with the administrator of the parents' wing before ten o'clock. I rang Rick first. Mary had arrived and Stephen was asleep. I hated dragging Rick in again, as if I couldn't do my share of watching without his being there, but he said he'd come.

I went to the parents' wing then and the supervisor brought me to a room at the end of a ward, not actually in the parents' wing. That was so that, if they needed to call us during the night, they wouldn't have to go through the ward to get to us. I told her my husband might be staying now as well and very obligingly she went off to look for a camp bed to put in the room.

I knew Sr Anna wanted to see me so I went back up to the Intensive Care waiting-room yet again. On the way I met one of James's nurses. She stopped to say hello to me and ask for him. Her demeanour was quite different from that of the night before.

Everyone was different now. No one expressed even a trace of optimism. She advised me that if James did go I should remember that there had been good times; there really had been a lot of good times! Sr Anna came up to the waiting-room. She'd ordered tea and it came on a tray. I asked her if there was any hope at all. She told me no. I believed her. I think from then I began to feel the end would not be very long away. That he would 'go' the following day. No one ever says 'die' in Crumlin.

Sr Anna, whom I had so resented the first time I met her – or rather the fixed attitudes I had assumed she would represent, and whom I had grown to so admire over the months – was now preparing me for the end of it all, regretting James's losing the fight after all he'd been through.

I asked her how she managed, how she kept going. She said it was often hard, dealing with very sick children, but that it was the love that kept her up. The love of the parents for their children, the love the children themselves, so very often special people in their own right, generated in their families. She said there was so much love shown between these walls that people outside would just not credit it. Sr Anna calmed me. I told her Rick was coming and that we were going to hold James.

I told her how angry I had been and how I used to take it out on God, give out to him. I was surprised, even then, how understanding she was. I can't remember her exact words but she more or less told me that was OK, that God would understand. She also referred, with praise, to us and the fact that we had visited James every day, day in, day out, regardless. I knew it was Rick's steadfastness and strength that had kept me going on that routine. I would have buckled under it several times had it not been for him. His sheer compassion and the depth of his concern and love for James made it unthinkable that we could let him down if it was humanly possible not to.

I still felt guilty, though, that I had not loved James enough. I had not accepted him. I had always wanted him to die, not to survive, not to grow up so different from the norm in a cruel world. Now that it was happening I felt even worse, and yet I didn't want him to go on as he was. I didn't want him to live much longer like this. I didn't know how long we could watch him like this. Yet I knew we'd have to, and would, until the end.

Sr Anna said she would come in to see James with me. As I was getting near his place my heart began to beat most erratically so that I was afraid it wasn't going to go back to its normal beat. I had to be helped into a chair feeling really stupid, as if I must look as if I was going to faint. It was the stress, I suppose, combined with exhaustion. After a few moments I was able to talk, say I was all right, look at James and cry again.

When Rick came we went straight back up to ICU. James's nurse asked us if we would like to have James confirmed. She told us that babies are not given the Sacrament of the Sick but can be confirmed if they are very ill. I vaguely remembered that from some religion class long ago. We said yes. I thought particularly of Rick's Mum and how she would like it – a special blessing. The chaplain was out but should be back by around half past ten. We decided to go ahead and hold James. The nurse suggested that we get a Babygro or something from his own clothes downstairs to dress him in. I ran downstairs. Again with a sense of urgency. I couldn't seem to slow down.

All his things – clothes, toys, activity centre, had been reduced to the contents of a black refuse sack. The nurse rummaged, picked out something, decided against it and then pulled out a soft Babygro that buttoned down the back and had animals on the front. It had been Stephen's and it was one I'd always liked. I took it. She closed the bag, all the time talking about James.

James's nurse had to pull back the sheet to try to put the Babygro on. From his waist to the top of his legs, James was just bandages. He was heartbreakingly swollen and it seemed to take all that was beautiful about him away, the things I had grown to love. And his eyes, those vital, expressive eyes, were shut.

I knew the nurse was trying to do this with dignity, to give us our baby for a moment to hold as if he was still ours to hold, but it didn't work. The Babygro was awkward. It was almost impossible to put on because of all the bandages and the drips. For me it just accentuated how much things had deteriorated from the situation in Special Care. This child could not be dressed. Our baby was joined to too much technology, swollen too big for his little frame.

Then they had to take off the ventilator and put on the manual breathing pump – a second nurse was helping – with a second or two gap at the changeover. That gap, I supposed, was the danger to his life. That nurse was pumping breath into him. When the time came to lift him – another danger to him – they picked up all the paper under him as well. Rick was nearest so he was given James to hold first. He broke down as as the unconscious body of our dying child was given to him. For Rick, I think, it was another stage in the realisation that he really was going to lose him. I was not sorry I had called him back into the hospital though, because this was important.

When I was given James I felt cheated because I felt I wasn't really being allowed to hold him properly. I don't know what I'd expected but with all those paper sheets I couldn't feel his warmth or the shape of his body or hold him close to me as you would naturally. We were allowed simply to hold him; they hadn't promised that we could cuddle him.

Time was limited too. He had to be laid down and put back on the ventilator. His heartbeat seemed steady still. There was no reaction from him. We went back to our usual way of putting one of our fingers into his fist. There was no reaction. He did not grip us at all.

We went back outside soon after. Out to that second floor landing. The stairs, the bench, the waiting-room. I felt it would not be days longer. I felt he would die the next day.

The next day was our wedding anniversary. Our third. We talked about that a bit; it had been on both our minds. We wondered if James would choose that day to give up.

The chaplain came back around eleven o'clock. James was back lying mostly motionless and unresponsive though there were occasional twitches and jerking movements too. His nurse told us he was no longer on the drug meant to stop all movement, but she said he was doing very little for himself.

James was anointed with chrism and blessed. It was a peaceful short ceremony. We were asked if we'd got our room sorted out. The nurses promised we would be called during the night if there was any change. We went down to the room, washed our teeth and got ready for bed. Bone tired.

Rick went to sleep quickly that night in the dark, unfamiliar bed. I had more difficulty this time. I was on the camp bed. Eventually I did fall asleep and slept for about three hours. Then woke again. Wide awake.

<u>13</u>

24 AUGUST

All that night I felt I was on call, alert, as if I should be there for James that night and never slip too far into sleep. I suppose I was over-tired, keyed up, a combination of many things. But it was a very long night. I was glad to have Rick there near me in the other bed but I felt it was my turn to watch over James and that it might well be the last time I would ever be able to.

When I couldn't lie still any more I got up and dressed and went back up to him. I don't remember the exact time but it was between three and four o'clock in the morning. The nurses seemed surprised to see me. His nurse asked if I'd like tea and went to get some. James was more or less the same as when we'd left him earlier.

The nurse minding the child beside him watched both of them now while his nurse was gone. And she talked to me. She said I must be very worried and asked if I'd slept at all. She said most parents managed to sleep through that part of the night anyway. She told me the little girl she was nursing had been in ICU for a week. Even though it was Intensive Care there were still personal touches: she had her own, beautiful, multi-coloured patchwork quilt over her and a musical teddy just like Stephen's. The nurse said that although she was very sick, at times she would wake up and smile and respond and liked that teddy to be played. The nurse said she was a lovely child.

My eyes went back to James. I asked the nurse if she had any children. She had one daughter.

James's nurse came back with the tea but I could hardly touch a drop. It seemed wrong, obscene almost, to take anything in front of James while he was lying there like that. The nurse pulled down the sheet to look at his abdomen. And for a clear moment I saw James as we had known him. His legs, because of the abnormality of his hips, lay splayed out a bit. They were just like that then, so characteristically and indisputably his, and his feet too, in their abnormality, pointing towards his head. It was comforting to see that something of his body was the same but awfully upsetting too.

I asked about the pads which had been put in on Monday night. The nurse said they couldn't be left in for more than forty-eight hours. I got the impression that she didn't think they would open him up again to take them out. Eventually I said I'd go back downstairs and try to sleep again. I left them watching over the children.

Rick hardly stirred but was aware of me coming back. I got into bed again. Eventually I dozed a bit but didn't sleep deeply. I think I got up again before six. I went to James again. Things were much the same as before. The nurse said she was sorry she could give me no more hope. It was still too early for anything. The hospital hadn't really woken up. I wandered downstairs to go to the toilet. I went along the quiet main corridor, past the shop and casualty, round into the coffee bar.

I went into the Ladies. I hated it. I splashed water on my face but you couldn't really wash there and it was too early to go down to the parents' wing. On my way back I met a porter at the main door. He'd a loud, gruff voice but was kindly.

'You don't, by any chance, own that car out there with the lights on, do you?' he asked. My heart sank. Not another problem. Which one? An orangey-red Fiesta?

'No, no. It mustn't be yours so. The one beside that – a blue one. The lights have been on all night. Battery'll be as flat as a pancake. It was like Blackpool illuminations here at half past ten last night. Lights left on. But we've no way of finding out who owns them, you know. We do our best but we've no way of telling.'

I ran out, looking into the car park. It was ours. The Nissan. Rick must have left the lights on when he arrived last night. It wouldn't have occurred to me that he might have. It was most unlike him. He never forgot things, was never scatterbrained like me. I had to get the keys and at least turn off the lights. I went back to our room and started rummaging. I had to disturb Rick slightly but got them and went back out. Of course there was no kick in the engine at all.

Then the dilemma of whether I should go home or stay started gnawing at me. I kept thinking of the previous morning and Stephen shunning us for having abandoned him. I couldn't bear the thought of that again and yet, could I leave James? How could I leave James? What if something happened? I was completely torn. Stephen might need me but it might be the last morning I could ever be with James. But then again I could be wrong. James might live another couple of days and for how many mornings could I leave Stephen?

I went back up to James. It was still awful to see him. Still a shock every single time. I asked his nurse what she thought. She said yes, why not go home. I could come back again then. They would ring me if anything at all happened and Rick would still be there. She said it was very hard for them, watching James as he was, so it must be absolutely harrowing for us. She touched his tummy gently with her fingers.

She said she didn't know what they would decide today. They might decide to turn off some more machines and things. We would have to wait and see. I asked when that was likely to be. She said they started doing their rounds about nine o'clock. Nothing would be done before then.

I decided then that I would go home to see Stephen for a little while.

James's nurse said she'd better say goodbye then. She said she'd hardly see us again. That was all but she was very definite. I hadn't the courage to ask her whether she was due on again that night. I put my finger through James's swollen hand. There was no reaction. I left him with his nurse and went back downstairs to Rick.

It was about seven o'clock by then and he was starting to wake up. I sat on the side of his bed. I said I'd go home if that was all right. He said he'd have to get the AA for the car. I told him all James's nurse had said and that I'd leave Stephen to the baby-minder's and the car to my father, and come back in later in a taxi so that we could go home together. He said he'd ring me. It was our wedding anniversary.

I went out into the bright, clear, early morning and got into the Fiesta. It was just after a quarter past seven. Once I began driving I really wanted to be home before Stephen got up so that he wouldn't know I'd deserted him again. I concentrated on getting home.

There was very little traffic. It was ten to eight when I opened the front door and immediately I heard voices. In the kitchen, Mary was talking to Stephen and he was sitting up in the high chair quite happily in his sleeping suit. I was relieved and glad to see him. Mary said they'd only been up a few minutes and that he'd been fine so far. We had our breakfast and got dressed, taking our time. Neither of us was in a rush, yet I kept looking up at the clock wondering when Rick would ring. We played with Stephen, then he followed Mary upstairs and watched her putting on her make-up, fascinated by all the jars and tubes.

At last Rick rang. He said the doctors had been around to see James and though the nurses wanted the ventilator turned off the doctors had said that was out of the question. He said the AA had come out and got the car going straight away.

Mary and I decided to walk down to the minder's. I thought a bit of air might do me good. Probably because I was so tired I seemed to be moving and thinking more slowly than usual. I walked back up home and got cheese, apples and biscuits for our lunch. Then I went back upstairs and got the little embroidered tunic that a friend of ours had sent as a present for James. It was still in its plastic bag, never worn. It was near enough to eleven o'clock by then.

I drove down to my father's house, about a mile away, had tea and phoned for a taxi. I rang the hospital again – the familiar number – and asked for Intensive Care. The nurse told me they had turned down the ventilator, that they would see how James did. I think she asked if I was coming in. She definitely said: 'Your husband is expecting you.' I asked her to tell him I was just waiting for a taxi and would be there as soon as I could. I had the feeling of urgency again.

The taxi came about ten minutes later. I felt very tense. The ventilator had been turned down. My husband was expecting me. The nurse had sounded both urgent and not urgent. Was it me reading between the lines? I couldn't restrain myself from asking the taxi driver to hurry. I nearly threw the money at him when we got to the steps of Crumlin. I ran up the two flights of stairs, plastic bag in hand. I rang the bell, washed my hands, put on the apron. Rick was in with James. He was still twitching a little. The heart monitor was bleeping away.

How was he?

The same. The ventilator down.

We stayed a few minutes. Then Rick said perhaps we should go and have some lunch. I said I had brought some stuff from home. He asked me about Stephen. We made another move to go out and then the nurse came over to us and said they were going to move James into a room on his own. She said it would give us more privacy. We stood up. They began, as on the previous night, preparing to disengage the ventilator momentarily and 'bag' him again. Three nurses were around him. We began to move in procession, the drip stands following the bed. I put my finger one more time into the little, swollen hand and it grasped mine – a clear, definite clasp of my finger – life! The open bed swung round the corner, one nurse pumping.

James was installed in the room the boy who'd had the heart operation had vacated. The bed was pushed into place. I looked up at the new heart monitor. It hadn't been connected yet. The ventilator was reconnected. James's lungs continued to rise and fall, mechanically. I looked up at the heart monitor again. Still nothing, and a third time. Nothing. I was about to point that out to the nurse. She had her finger on James's pulse. But as I opened my mouth to speak she said, 'He's going.'

Just that. The monitor was connected but there was no heartbeat.

'His heart's going,' she said.

Rick and I spoke together. James, James we love you. We told him over and over.

James was dead.

It was 24 August 1988. Our third wedding anniversary. A quarter to one.

Very quickly James was disconnected from all the the tubes,

drips and the ventilator. His nurse picked him up, wrapped him in a blanket and handed him, still warm, to us. For the first time in three days we were really allowed to hold our child but he was our dead child now. He did look peaceful. We just sat there, holding him for I don't know how long.

Almost all the nurses from Special Care came up to see us after a while, to be in the room with us and James's body. All but one of them was in tears. We found ourselves comforting the nurses. They had all been James's mothers, had all loved him. It was a tribute to his little person that they had loved him so much.

Later, I gave them the tunic to dress James in. The social worker came up and kissed his forehead. She asked us if we had considered donating anything – she said only James's eyes would really be suitable, but if we wanted . . .

My immediate reaction was no, please leave him alone now. He's suffered enough. I knew he was dead and yet I didn't because I couldn't bear the thought of anyone doing anything else awful to him and yet now it was only his body that was there so it wouldn't have mattered. The social worker said that was fine and if it had been mentioned to us sooner perhaps it would have been better, that it was difficult to decide this now. I've always regretted that we didn't give his eyes to another child.

The nurses allowed us to use the station in ICU to make a couple of phone calls. First I asked Rick to throw out the food that I had had with me when he died. Then we made calls – to my father, Rick's mother, Margaret and Don and the babyminder. Of course she wouldn't tell Stephen but somehow I wanted her, who was minding Stephen, to know that he no longer had a little brother on this earth.

14

AFTERWARDS

Ciaran and the chaplain concelebrated the Mass of the Holy Angels for James in the hospital chapel where he had been christened.

We brought his little white coffin in our car out to County Wicklow and buried James's body under the shadow of the Sugarloaf mountain, beside his great-grandmother.

On the day James died Siamese twins were born in the Coombe Hospital, Katie and Eilish. Katie died in April 1992 after an operation to separate the twins.

It hurt the first time I heard another mother, a complete stranger, calling her son James to sit down.

A famine report on the news showed a hollow-faced black baby, all eyes and skull, suffering from malnutrition. He was six months old, the reporter said. He was almost exactly the same weight as James had been a few days before he died.

Eight months later my father was knocked down crossing the road. He died four months later without ever regaining consciousness.

Eight months after that my mother died in her sleep in the early hours of the morning of my father's birthday.

Two weeks later our third child, Aengus, was born. A healthy baby boy, he weighed in at 3.6 kilos.

15

MARY

Why did I write this book? Well, it was good for me to write it all down but I could have done that privately. The reason I went beyond that and sought a publisher was that I know I am not alone in the very mixed-up feelings I had towards our second child. I know other mothers who have had children with disabilities, whether mental or physical, have had ambivalent feelings also, have at times felt they hated their own children. They have even wished they would die and have then suffered the awful guilt that comes with those feelings.

This book would never have come into existence if James had lived. I would never have publicised his disabilities then, for fear of hurting him in some way. Neither would I have wanted to say, publicly, that I'd wished, when he was born, that he would disappear off the face of the earth. Because he is no longer with us I am freer to speak and hope that other parents can identify with what I'm saying and, perhaps, feel less guilty or less abnormal as a result.

I also think that modern medicine poses a lot of moral dilemmas about how actively very ill children should be treated, when one should finally call a halt, when it becomes more humane to allow someone to die. Medical expertise has advanced so quickly that most of us have little or no idea of the implications and only think about them when we're faced with a decision about a loved one.

The Third World also haunts me. I remember how nothing at all was spared in the care of James and then I think of Ethiopia, Somalia, Rwanda, where perfectly healthy children are dying because there's no food. The world seems topsy-turvy, to say the least of it.

I am a different person now compared with when I first got married. James did change me. I had to face up to the ugly side of me, the basic instincts that are part of me and the negative, selfish emotions that emerged when I was put under severe stress. It was a long, long time before I allowed myself even to mourn him and to see that, as well as the bad feelings, I had also learned to love him. I suppose it took me a long time to forgive myself. If he had lived it would have taken me years longer because I would also have been struggling with day-to-day existence, the ups and downs, more surgery, hope, disappointment. But I have had the luxury of time to think and space to put between me and the situation. I know that parents who are still struggling may think it's all very well for me to talk. It *is* easy for me compared with them and there is also the danger of sentimentalising the situation and seeing it in a rosy glow from this distance. It was always going to be hard. I still believe it was probably for the best that James only spent a short time here. At least he did know moments of happiness and he never realised what was wrong with him. He was showered with love by many people and I know no one can harm or hurt him any more now.

He is a part of my life and always will be. Sometimes, when I look at my two beautiful sons, their heads bent over a book, or when they're running down to the sea, I feel the absence of James, the missing child, like a shadow between them and like a pain inside. Then I wonder would he ever have been well enough to go to the beach and run into the sea himself. Life isn't black and white. I suppose I've learnt to accept the grey too, the shades of feelings, of meanings, of right and wrong and to accept the grey in myself, while trying my best to rise above it.

I am stronger, though. I know I can face almost anything, knowing what I've already gone through. It puts everything into perspective. My job, while still important to me, is no longer something I cling to. I know I could survive without it if I had to. People are more important, are the most important. I have learnt how precious life really is. If James did nothing else, he taught me how very lucky I am to have two healthy children, how miraculous and beautiful and perfect they are. And I go on realising that with an intensity which doesn't seem to dim. I know how very lucky I am and it is a gift to have been shown that and to know it so surely.

16

RICK

I remember the night that James was born, a doctor telling me that he would be taken to Crumlin hospital in an ambulance. At that time, I had no idea where Crumlin was, so I followed the ambulance through the quiet night streets, with snow beginning to fall. It all felt unreal, as I concentrated on driving with so many other thoughts and feelings going through my mind. At the hospital, I was told to wait in the corridor while James was settled in Special Care and a doctor called to see him. I waited there for a couple of hours, with little to do since it was night time and there was no one around. About 2 a.m. I could wait no longer and went into Special Care to see if I could find anyone. Much later I would confidently go in and out of the ward without a second thought but at that time I had no idea of procedures or protocol. A nurse told me apologetically that they'd forgotten I was there and that the doctor had been and gone. So began many months of uncertainty and turmoil, but also, some lasting memories and happy occasions.

For the first few weeks, with the uncertainty of James's sex and the question of whether or not he would survive, I seemed to get by in a state of automation. On the one hand I was rather detached and rational, able to respond to the questions we were asked and carry out day-to-day activities fairly normally. On the other, I had just switched off, I think, from the pressure of too much information that I couldn't comprehend. I knew that I had a few clear things to do, the main one being to try to support Mary as she was struggling to come to terms with the situation. I also wanted to protect Stephen from too much distress and to see what would happen with James. The rest could wait.

And that was one of the main differences between Mary and me: how we coped with the situation we were thrown into. All along, she, with her concern as a mother, would worry about the long-term implications of James's condition. How would he cope if he were brought up as a girl? What would others' reaction to him be? It wasn't that I wasn't concerned with these questions too, but to me they were too remote. For another day. For now, what mattered was getting through the next few days and weeks, whichever they happened to be.

It's true that a father's role is seen as to be strong and to provide support in situations beyond a family's control. And that's what I felt I should do, especially in the early weeks. And I wanted to do it, too. It gave me a clear role, something to do instead of being paralysed by the uncertainty that surrounded us. That was the positive side. The less positive side was that I didn't allow myself really to explore or come to terms with what was happening. While Mary was being hit by waves of conflicting and strong emotions, I was to some extent stepping back from what was going on.

The first weeks were a real immersion in hospital life and a lesson on the way decisions on a person's future are made. As Mary has said, we had some difficulty in reconciling our own views with those of the professionals at times. The most important thing for us, though, was that we talked over our own position, reflected on what we had been told and stuck together on whatever course of action we felt was for the best. If the decision had been to bring James up as a girl, I don't know what we would have done, as this was so unbelievable to us both. But thankfully that was one issue we didn't have to face in the end.

But what about James? At first, I found it difficult to think of him as a real person. I knew he was our child and that his future was uncertain but because of his problems, he *seemed* ours only in some intangible way. As he got over the first operation and the problems he had following that, he grew to be more one of the family to me. I'll certainly never forget his smile. His eyes used to light up, and as his smile widened, it spread all around him. He was certainly a bright child and full of curiosity whenever anything new came into his limited environment. I'd often wonder what it was like for him, living all the time in a hospital incubator or bed, confined to stimulus from a small area and circle of people. But at least the stimulus he got was a loving one. The nurses treated him as an individual, someone they obviously cared for, and that helped us a lot.

The middle period of his life was one that settled into some kind of routine for us. While working, visiting James and looking after Stephen at home was physically very tiring, at least it gave us a routine of sorts. In many ways I found this time the easiest to cope with. While the problems were still there in the background, they were something that did not need immediate attention. I could welcome each stage in James's development and deal with each minor setback, in much the same way as with another child. Of course, the situation was very different, but I tried not to think too much of that. I also felt less need to consider how Mary was coping and just let things move along as well as they could. The highlights, wheeling James around the hospital, the couple of times we got to bring him home and his christening were all special.

Though very ordinary things in themselves, they took on an extraordinary dimension thanks to our circumstances.

Crumlin Hospital was a part of our lives by this time. We were dealing on a daily basis with a world that had been foreign to us just a few short months before. At times I find it hard to believe that it is still central to so many parents' and children's lives now. As a hospital it has a role in healing where possible, and caring for all. Yet in a very real sense it also becomes a centre for all sorts of other hopes and feelings too. In the case of James, I know that much of his spirit resides in the walls of the hospital, just as it lives with us wherever we are.

James's second, and last, major operation was a time of mixed feelings. I was anxious that he should come through it and that it should not take too much out of him. But at the same time, I knew that I didn't want him to suffer too much. If it was better for him that he didn't pull through, I was hoping that it would happen quickly and peacefully. In the event, neither of these eventualities were to happen. I still remember the time between his operation and his death as a very difficult one. From the time that the surgeon had told us that there was no hope, I too had no hope of his pulling through. Yet, stubborn character that he was, he hung on. I found it difficult to be with him in Intensive Care. The baby that was there drugged and motionless on the bed wasn't the James that I knew and loved. I was glad of the chance to get out and then I felt guilty for not being with him . . . There was no solution to this.

To some extent roles were reversed now. Mary was stronger than me and supportive of me at this time, much as I was of her in the earlier times. We have been lucky in this. Usually one of us was able to summon up the strength to carry on when the other wasn't capable any more. This happened throughout James's life and was central to helping us get through. By the time of his death, we had both done our share of supporting and being supported. The last moments were for James, as the love that had grown between us all provided the means to ease his passage.

Of course the death and funeral were extremely sad and difficult. Yet the help of family, friends and colleagues from work helped through a time when I found myself as if in a state of shock, doing most things automatically. Mentally, I didn't find it too difficult to cope. I had always hoped that James would pull through but above that I had always wanted what was best for him. If that meant a short life, then so be it. Physically, though, I found the aftermath of James's death difficult. Your body can keep going for so long when it has to. But when you relax, all the accumulated wear and tear hits hard. And that's what happened to me. It took a long time for me to get back to feeling myself again.

And looking back now at James's life and death? I don't really want to rationalise it by trying to find meanings for why he was here and the problems he had. To me that doesn't make much sense. Rather, I know that for someone who was here for such a little time he had a big impact on those around him. Like a pebble dropped into a pool, the ripples he created continue to grow and have a hidden depth. Not only have Mary and I been affected – and Stephen – but also our families and friends. James's life was a challenge to us all in different ways and one that continues its influence. I don't really feel that I want to grieve for him, or wish for the childhood that he never had. I feel that his life carried its own meaning, whatever it was, and that now it's up to us to enrich and develop the memories we have of that time.

Not that all the memories are happy ones or ones that we can be proud of. Far from it. But they were and are real and strong, and in their own way a testimony to James. It's not as if he or we are special people in any way. We are ordinary people who were thrown into an extraordinary situation. Like many parents who have to cope with the illness of a child, all we could do is face it as honestly as we could. And in telling his story, Mary has tried to express the thoughts and feelings that accompany such a situation. To me, it's a way of expressing that it's all right and natural to feel contradictory emotions and unwanted feelings. Life is like that. I don't know if I'm a better or a worse person for having gone through what we did. To be honest, I don't feel much different. But I do carry the memories of James with me at all times, and to that extent my life is affected. Ultimately I feel proud that we as a family continue to grow and behave just like most families do. Not because of, or even despite, James. But he's there – a part of us – and always will be.

And finally. We have two boys, Stephen and Aengus, who are a great source of pride and happiness. Not to mention frustration, annoyance and tiredness! And I have Mary. We've been through so much together, and have come through together. I feel that she's been hard on herself in telling this story, honest about her feelings, but she also gave and gives so much. But that is obvious, I think.

And we have James.

14

LETTERS II

August 25

My dear Mary and Rick

Words cannot express a lot at times like this but we feel so much for you all. It is everyone's sorrow that James didn't make it, but Our Blessed Lord knows what was best for him and you and you now have someone to intercede for you in Heaven.

I had a sister of ten months, who died five months before I was born, and in times of stress I often asked her help.

It's lovely that you have Stephen to console you. Your Daddy and Denise tell me what a wonderful little lad he is.

You have both been through a very stressful time, so I hope you will have a little holiday for the three of you, while there is a chance of some fine weather. I am sure Stephen will keep you happy and busy.

Much love and prayers

Auntie Babby

[my godmother]

September 4

Dear Mary and Rick

I was so very very sorry to hear about poor little James. This must be a really terrible time for you both especially after all the worry and trauma you've been through over the last seven months. Although I'm sure you feel you at least had the consolation of knowing James for seven months you must feel his loss all the more having had this time with him.

My prayers and sympathy go to you both. I do so hope that in time the pain of his loss will be easier to bear.

I am thinking of you all the time and praying that you will find the strength to get through this very difficult time.

Love to you both and to Stephen

from

Paula

September 19

Dear Mary and Rick

I was both saddened and relieved to hear from Denise that James had finally given in and passed peacefully away.

Words can hardly express how your friends at Dulwich Runners feel for you all at this every sad time in your lives. Life is hard to understand at times and James came into this world with a purpose to fulfil. What that was you may not be able to think of at this time but in a few years you will look back and realise what he taught you.

You are with us in our thoughts and prayers and we look forward to seeing you in Dulwich very soon.

Much love

Sue, Chris and family